"A step-by-step how-to guide on building meaningful connections for every stage of life! From the delivery driver at your local market to family and friends, they are all part of your village. In *Build Your Village*, Florence gives you the tools that will enhance your life."

Douglas E. Noll, author of *De-Escalate* and *Elusive Peace*

"Easy to digest, informative, and valuable—Florence Ann Romano's *Build Your Village* is redefining the age-old phrase 'It takes a village.'"

Joseph Fatheree, NEA National Award for Teaching Excellence 2009 and Illinois Teacher of the Year 2007

"As Florence Ann Romano brilliantly points out in *Build Your Village*, community is a necessity to life—and we have the ability to create our own. Be true to yourself, reassess your values (and what you value in others), and infuse your life with support and compassion."

Michael Clinton, former president and publishing director of HEARST Magazine, founder of ROAR Forward, and author of *ROAR*

"Yes, it does take a village, but with gut checks, exercises, and action steps, *Build Your Village* from Florence Ann Romano makes identifying your community easier than you think. This is the go-to guide for anyone who has ever felt disconnected."

Bridgetta Tomarchio, celebrity publicist, book coach, and mom

"Florence Ann Romano's *Build Your Village* reminds me of the richness that others bring to our lives, as well as the value that we contribute to theirs."

Barry Shore, The Ambassador of Joy™ and host of *The Joy of Living* podcast

Build Your Village

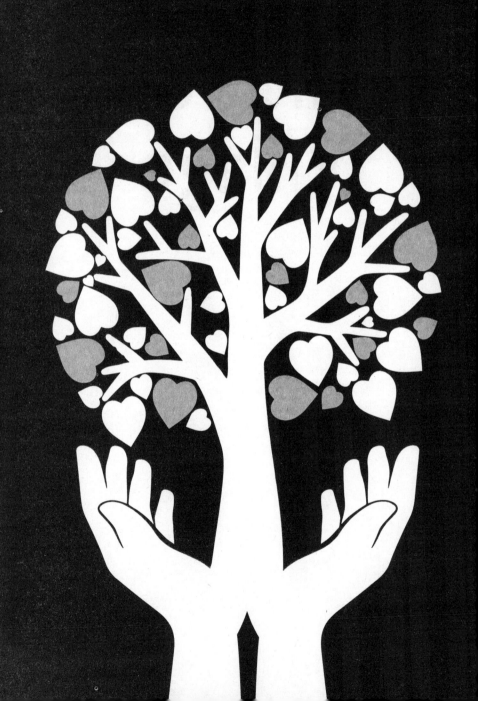

Build Your Village

A Guide to Finding Joy and Community in Every Stage of Life

Florence Ann Romano

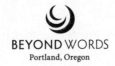

BEYOND WORDS
Portland, Oregon

BEYOND WORDS

1750 S.W. Skyline Blvd., Suite 20
Portland, Oregon 97221-2543
503-531-8700 / 503-531-8773 fax
www.beyondword.com

First Beyond Words paperback edition February 2023

All names, locations, and identifying details have been changed to protect the privacy of individuals.

For more information about special discounts for bulk purchases, please contact Beyond Words Special Sales at 503-531-8700 or specialsales@beyondword.com.

Managing editor: Lindsay Easterbrooks-Brown
Editors: Michele Cohn, Bailey Potter, Alison Lowenstein
Copyeditor: Ashley Van Winkle, Emmalisa Sparrow Wood
Proofreader: Linda M. Meyer
Illustration: Annalise Batista
Design: Sara E. Blum
Composition: William H. Brunson Typography Services

Manufactured in the United States of America

10 9 8 7 6 5 4 3 2 1

Library of Congress Cataloging-in-Publication Data:

Names: Romano, Florence Ann, author.
Title: Build your village : a guide to finding joy and community in every
   stage of life / Florence Ann Romano.
Description: Portland, Oregon : Beyond Words, [2023]
Identifiers: LCCN 2022035845 (print) | LCCN 2022035846 (ebook) |
   ISBN 9781582708867 (paperback) | ISBN 9781582708874 (ebook)
Subjects: LCSH: Social groups. | Communities. | Social interaction |
   Social psychology.
Classification: LCC HM716 .R65 2023 (print) | LCC HM716 (ebook) |
   DDC 302—dc23/eng/20220818
LC record available at https://lccn.loc.gov/2022035845
LC ebook record available at https://lccn.loc.gov/2022035846

The corporate mission of Beyond Words Publishing, Inc.: *Inspire to Integrity*

*To Nana and Mom . . . my soft landing, my role models,
the loves of my life. We share the same shadow. Within that
shadow, you showed me the village.*

Contents

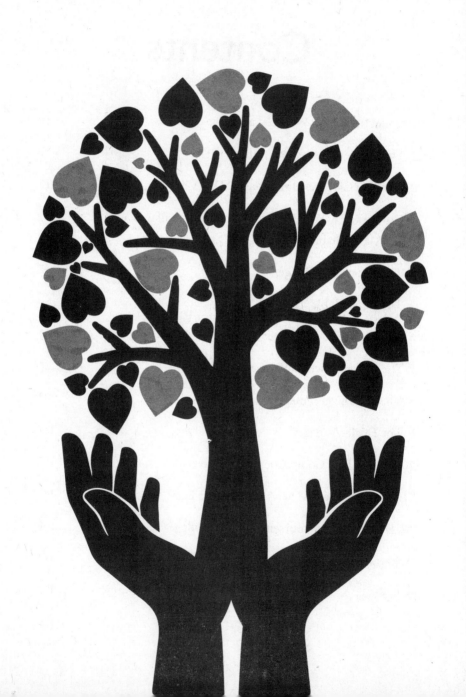

Introduction

Why We Need a Village

Humans are social creatures. It's a phrase we hear time and time again, but rarely do we process the magnitude of it. Just as we need water, air, food, and shelter, we need community. The former needs are more concrete and more easily acquired. Water, food, and shelter can all be purchased, and luckily, air is free. But where do we find community? Sometimes we are fortunate enough to be born into it, but oftentimes we must build our own. This is easier said than done, and as a result, a loneliness epidemic plagues our country. We don't always take loneliness as seriously as we should—it can cause our bodies major physical harm. The CDC cited a recent study that found "social isolation significantly increased a person's risk of premature death from all causes, a risk that may rival those of smoking, obesity, and physical inactivity," and "loneliness was associated with higher rates of depression, anxiety, and suicide."[1]

In order to live happy, healthy, and full lives, we need to tend to our social health just as much as we tend to our physical health. But how do we do it? We've all heard the popular African proverb, "It takes a village to raise a child." The phrase has been uttered countless times by politicians, authors, and probably even people you know. There's always someone touting the merits of the "village." Michelle Obama remarked, "It truly takes a village to raise children. Build your village wherever you are. It will be your salvation and keep you sane."[2] But the real question is, how do we get directions to reach (or build) this village? And is this an exclusive community reserved solely for parents of young children? Would I be allowed in if I wasn't a raising a child?

Although the phrase is "it takes a village to raise a child," this shouldn't be a reward for having children. *Everyone* needs a village. We can't do everything ourselves, and being social is vital for our survival.[3] The United States has been dealing with the catastrophic results of our increasingly isolated lifestyles. The consequences of being lonely are dire—The Health Resources and Services Administration states that loneliness can increase the risk of dementia by 50 percent.[4]

This means having trustworthy friends is an essential component to staying healthy. No matter what stage of life you're in, it's beneficial to have a group of supportive people around you. Being surrounded by people who care helps both your physical and mental well-being. Of course, anyone who has dreaded spending Thanksgiving with their family might disagree. It's true we can't choose our families, but we can choose the people we surround ourselves with. And after reading this book, you might even be able to isolate and analyze certain traits in your family members to see how you can better fit into one another's lives.

You may be surprised to learn that a number of the people you thought were providing you with love and support are not actually serving as essential members of your community. This was the hard truth I had to acknowledge—just because you have a ton of plans and scores of people in your life doesn't mean you have a village.

This book aims to make the distinction between a group of people and a *community* of people. A village comprises people who help one another out. This means people with a calendar filled with plans would benefit from taking a meaningful look at the relationships in their lives and how their actions impact other people. Having a large social circle doesn't mean you have a community.

There is a myriad of instances in life when we must rely on this thoughtfully curated group of people, and there are numerous villages we can create—from makeshift ones at a moment of crisis to more concrete ones that help us in the everyday. And each of these communities can help us get through difficult times, tackle challenges, and celebrate moments of triumph. Most importantly, having this team means you don't have to do everything on your own, which makes things easier.

For more than a decade I was known as The Windy City Nanny. I had a web series where I brought awareness to the role communities play in families' lives.[5] I also wrote a children's book, *Nanny and Me*, because I felt there wasn't a book that addressed the role of a caregiver in a child's life. Writing this book established me as a childcare advocate, and I've since been invited to more than five hundred media engagements, including national talk shows and news segments, where I've discussed village and childcare advocacy. Then I pivoted from nannying and spent more than a decade running Kindred Content, a purpose-driven video production company that worked with nonprofits and brands to create digital content. Creating meaningful content was endlessly fulfilling, and if you've ever been part of a production team, you know the importance of a village.

However, it was when I was a nanny that I was part of multiple families' support systems, and I was able to identify six types of villagers one should have in a complete working village. After study-ing and interviewing people in numerous communities I was a part of, I discovered the six essential traits that one needs to form a com-munity of consciously compassionate people. This doesn't mean you need to rush out and find six people to add to your friend group, but it does mean we should approach our relationships thoughtfully. Curating a group of people who have specific traits that complement one another is the key to building this world.

Even if you're a person who is a bit more introverted, you can still utilize and be part of a village. You have the option of choosing each villager's intensity level and how much you can give to the commu-nity. Even small moments, like sending a message of encouragement or donating food when someone is struggling can help you create a legacy of kindness.

The village might not always look the way you want. For instance, we all remember having our lives transformed from being in-person to online during the COVID-19 pandemic. Back then, some of us even branched out and created a global digital village during that isolating time, which proves that your community can consist of any caring people rather than only those who are close in proximity. It's not the distance but the dedication of each person that matters. This means that even if you're alone, you don't have to be lonely. This book will help you learn the language to communicate with others so you will be able to construct a life where you feel you're both cared for and also able to care for others.

Like the global pandemic, there will be times when we discover everything has fallen apart for reasons beyond our control, and though this might be hard to admit, sometimes we sabotage our own lives. Whatever the reason, you can work to rebuild or redefine your village. During my years of establishing multiple communities,

I've developed instructions on how to create one. There are specific qualities that we need to find in others and foster in ourselves to create a community that nurtures us and helps us grow.

Pete Seeger said, "I want to turn the clock back to when people lived in small villages and took care of each other."[6] This is a dream many of us share, but as a country we are more disconnected than ever. Learning how to foster certain characteristics in yourself that have the potential to help others is the first step to learning to let love in. Once you can do this, you'll discover deeper relationships with the people in your lives and will stave off the serious side effects of loneliness.

This book aims to demystify the notion of community and help you build lasting relationships with those in your life. With gut-check questions to guide you as you build your support system and action steps to help you establish the foundation of the village, this book serves as a step-by-step guide on how to build, strengthen, and maintain your new worlds. If you're wondering what "gut-check" questions are, they are questions that make you reflect on how you address certain situations in your life. Asking yourself tough questions and taking inventory of your life is essential to your well-being and emotional growth. We need to reflect on our past actions to successfully move forward into the future. This is why I paired the questions with the action steps, because once we've discovered patterns we've followed in the past, we can take steps to change our behavior. The action steps are little steps we can take to make big changes in our lives.

This type of journey involves self-reflection, as the concept of a village means something different to all of us. I've created a series of quick quizzes and exercises within each chapter to help you define what *village* means to you. I suggest that you set aside a notebook or electronic document to journal in, so that you can document all the work you're doing to help construct your community.

As you embark on this journey of creation, be patient with yourself. This book will give you all the tools you need to create a village, even if it takes a little while. Just like in a garden, the seeds of the community you plant need a little tending, but soon they begin to sprout.

The Importance of Your Village

The Value of Community

Alone we can do so little. Together we can do so much.
Helen Keller

Take a moment to think about the different relationships in your life. From your best friend to your barista, there are more than you'd think—people with whom you interact and by whom your life is shaped. You probably have categories that you subconsciously divide these people into: your family, your besties, your coworkers, your casual acquaintances, and I'm sure a ton more. You probably don't question these implicit divisions—and why would you? They are part of your everday life. *Community* is a word that gets thrown around a lot, from community outreach to community theater, but few of us really understand what it means to be an active member of a loving and supportive community.

My understanding of community didn't develop overnight. It's a culmination of my many years as a care provider. However, one particularly poignant moment that I recall is the day a young mother handed me her baby daughter. As she did, I noticed the mother had tears in her eyes. Though this is typical of mothers leaving their children for the first time, in this woman, I saw a sparkle, because she trusted someone to watch her baby (me!) and could go back to work to provide for her family. Although she had older children whom she had stayed home with as infants, she accepted that, at this stage in her life, she needed help to make her dreams possible.

A few weeks later, I took her older daughter to her first tennis lesson. As I sat with the mothers, they asked me about my "daughter."

"I'm the nanny," I explained, worrying that it might create a barrier between us. However, the mothers were accepting, and they integrated me into their group. I felt like I was taking a "mommy master class." As I observed them, I began to a notice a pattern— each was constantly crediting other people for helping them with their children. This isn't to say that they were self-deprecating or were diminishing their own roles in the lives of their children but rather that they were celebrating the villages they had each created.

Once I was accepted into those mothers' worlds, I studied how their villages worked. Within a short while, I had constructed my own, consisting of nannies and other parents. I'll admit that this idea—creating a community that works to help one another—was a concept I used when I transitioned to my new career in digital content, as well as in my personal life. Yes, I took everything I learned in the trenches as a nanny. (Okay, I wasn't exactly "in the trenches," but I was frequently standing near germ-infested ball pits, and there was never a day that I didn't come home with stained clothes.)

I noticed that this family I worked for, like the moms I had befriended, had people in their lives who anticipated their needs, and the family did the same in return; from evening babysitting collectives to carpooling, they achieved balance by asking for help. Yet I also observed other families who socialized frequently but weren't thriving like the families who had a support system. I felt like I was an apprentice who was learning the secret to a balanced life. For years I took notes and watched how the families constructed support systems and utilized the people in their lives. During these years of observation and study, I realized that a great deal of the positive interactions I was witnessing could be boiled down to just three ingredients: build a village, let love in, and ask for help. Once we master these three skills, we can raise families, launch businesses, achieve goals, and find balance in this everchanging world.

If you've ever visited the home of someone with kids, you might be familiar with an ever-present piece of paper, usually well-worn, affixed to their refrigerator with a magnet picked up as a memento from one of their vacations. The paper has the pediatrician's number, the parents' cellphone numbers, and maybe one other emergency contact. Those are the essential numbers we need if something, God forbid, goes wrong, but that list seems rather barren. We need other people to help us when we're feeling challenged and to celebrate our happy moments with us.

I studied the families I worked for who appeared to seamlessly create a village. Whom were they bringing into their lives, and how did those relationships benefit everyone? And even though I wasn't a parent, how could I create my own village that could help me? And how could I be part of other people's villages?

I noticed that once these families established a community, they could navigate the chaotic years of parenting. But parenting isn't the only chaotic period in people's lives. I know my post-college years were filled with decision-making and rebuilding communities. I also realized by watching the parents build their villages that being part of a community isn't codependent—it's caring. When we reflect on our roles and others' roles in our lives, we understand the importance of friends and families, especially when we're organizing our lives.

Inspired by that ubiquitous contact list on the fridge, and observing the villages the tennis moms had constructed, I created a helpful tool for families who feel challenged by trying to find the right people to cultivate their own groups. It's a chart that guides them through the process of identifying people who can support them in different roles and then asking for their help. I featured this chart on my web series *Windy City Nanny*, and it was great to see how the simple act of casting the people in your life into helpful roles can transform an overwhelmed family. The family that was featured realized they weren't alone. They started to build their village, let love in, and ask for help.[1]

When I posted the chart on my blog, readers reached out to comment on how helpful it was.[2] Although families were thankful that I had created this village-building tool, I was equally thankful because I had drafted a blueprint for creating communities in every aspect of *my* life as well. It took me awhile to realize this, but when I did it was my inspiration for writing this book.

By this point in my life I had transitioned from a career in nannying to digital content and had established myself in Chicago. When I moved to the city, straying from my suburban roots (spoiler alert: I later made my way back to the suburbs), I knew few people in the city. The only person I could call on for help was my building's super.

I even—this is embarrassing—had to call him to help me zip up a dress. I realized that I needed a village.

Although I had a bunch of friends to have a glass of wine with after work, those were relationships based on small talk. Something you should know about me is I don't like small talk; I like real talk! Once you *really* talk with someone, you develop a deeper relationship with them. But how could I even meet someone I wanted to have a real talk with? And how could I casually slip into the conversation that I need their help assembling an office chair? I didn't want to ask the super for yet another favor—I was still recovering from the embarrassment of having to call him to zip up my dress.

In constructing my community, the roadblock I had to face was myself. I felt like I didn't deserve such support. I thought that because I wasn't raising a child, I didn't need that village. But a village shouldn't be your reward for having children. If you don't have children, you still deserve a support system!

This inspired me to go back to the drawing board with my chart. While tweaking the chart, I thought about the many other stages in life when having helpful people around is necessary. In fact, as I write this book, I am considering whether or not to become a single mother by choice. I am going through IVF to freeze my eggs! Each community looks a bit different, but they both offer consciously compassionate people.

You Don't Have to Do it Alone

I can't tell you how many things I've done to stay healthy while dealing with thyroid disease and undergoing in vitro fertilization (IVF). Clean living is essential. I've given up dairy (an act I'm fairly certain is considered illegal in the Midwest), I wake up before most of the Midwest to work out on my treadmill, and I limit my sugar intake. I know that people have to make a conscious choice to live a healthful life, but there are other factors that impact mortality besides keeping up with routine health exams and maintaining healthy nutritional habits. In the past few years, I've read countless articles about a loneliness epidemic. In fact, one piece said that being lonely is as bad as smoking almost a pack of cigarettes a day.[3]

We all know what it feels like to be alone in a new place. Every time you start a new job, class, or hobby, you might feel awkward and isolated despite being surrounded by people. This is a normal side effect of being in a transitional period in life. This is also healthy: it helps you grow and gives you the opportunity to learn about yourself and others.

On the flip side, my friends and family have guiltily confessed to me that they dream about having a day to spend alone, where they didn't have to interact with their children, spouse, or coworkers. Each time I heard this confession, I kept my mouth shut. I didn't want them to know I'd heard it before. This was their revelation, and I took the role of listener. But this feeling is normal; people need time alone to recharge. You don't have to be surrounded by people every waking minute of the day! I can't tell you how much I love having my own house and being able to walk around in PJs all weekend without any judgement.

While choosing to fly solo for one day can be a luxury in a harried life, living a life alone can damage a person's health. And it should be noted that you can also surround yourself with people and still feel lonely.

Remember, the beauty of having a village is that you can call upon your community to help you, but you can also help others. People will benefit from your company as much as you benefit from theirs.

What Type of People Do You Need in Your Village?

We all cast people into certain roles in our lives. We might not do this intentionally but subconsciously. We have the friend we love to watch reality TV with or the person we text when we're heading to the gym. This book will ask you to pay closer attention and question those roles. Throughout the book there will be exercises to help you develop deeper relationships with the types of people around you, as well as with yourself. However, before you start digging and questioning, I have a quick quiz for you to take. If you're on the hunt for new villagers to add to your life, these questions will help you vet potential candidates. It will also help you see if the people around you are worth keeping in your village!

Should This Person Be in My Village? "Vetting for the Village"

Ask yourself these three questions about the person you are considering inviting into your circle:

1 **Are they willing to listen?**

2 **Are they good at recognizing what you need?**

3 **Will they make you feel understood?**

7

These may sound like simple questions, but the answers seldom are. The answers will help you see if the people in your life make good members of your community. Perhaps some display uncompromising behaviors; they can't see past themselves and will therefore not truly see you. Question whether they are listening to you. This doesn't mean they agree with everything you're saying but are able to hear your needs and attempt to fulfill them. If you answered yes to all three questions, you have found someone who will enhance both your village and your life.

Once you find solid people to build a village with, this doesn't necessarily mean you're comfortable asking these people for help. Asking people to support you is challenging. When I was hosting my web series, plenty of parents on the show were reluctant to ask for help, for numerous reasons. Of course, I always stressed the importance of community, and they would repeat that they didn't want to bother other people or that they were chronically overwhelmed and therefore believed they couldn't help others. I reassured them that people don't join a community because they expect someone to reciprocate. They join a community because they care. So, in the simplest of terms, the type of people one needs are caring people. But here's the really important part: not everyone cares in the same way.

I remember ages ago when a girlfriend gave me a copy of the book *The Five Love Languages* by Gary Chapman.[4] I wondered what all the hoopla about the book was and, I'll admit, I was suspicious of it. Then I read it, and it was powerful. I had never thought of defining love that way. If we figured out the love language our partners were speaking and what dialect, we could communicate more effectively. But rather than only using the information from that book to define my love language with romantic partners, I started studying how all the people in my life communicated their love, because the same concept applies to caring. Everyone speaks their own language when it comes to caring. Each person has a certain set of traits that is beneficial to the village and helps it run smoothly.

In this book I'll outline qualities for six essential villagers. Before you have a meltdown trying to find six actual people to populate your village, note that people can fulfill multiple roles. I suggest you have at least three people in your circle, though. I must warn you not to depend on only one person to fulfill all the characteristics of a village, because doing so would be overwhelming and might damage your relationship.

Whom do you need in your village? You need a variety of people who bring a multitude of skills that help others. For instance, my dad can't change a lightbulb. My mom is the one with the toolkit and will repair anything, but my father dispenses invaluable business advice and never steered me in the wrong direction when I was running my own business.

If you feel guilty when you ask for help, I want you to know that people want to help others. If you're cynical, you might not believe me, but I have proof. Have you ever seen one of those GoFundMe pages that went viral? They are filled with donations from strangers who are trying to help in whatever way they can. If you let your wall down, put your pride aside, jump over the hurdles, and ask for help, you will achieve a deeper sense of community and will cultivate more meaningful relationships.

How do you find your first villager? It starts with you. Ask someone if *they* need help with something. One of my best girlfriends and sorority sister (Go Pi Beta Phi!) was at the end of her pregnancy when she disclosed to me that it would be difficult to run her business when the baby arrived. I promised that I'd watch the baby one day a week. After she had the baby, she reached out and asked me if that offer was still on the table. (Let's be honest, we all make blanket promises we don't intend to keep.) I told her I was honored to be the person she trusted with her baby. I watched the baby once a week for six months. She was able to get work done, and now I have a bond with her daughter. Another way I help is by reaching out to friends via text. There's one friend I send a weekly text, which reads "Wellness check." She responds by unloading what happened that week. It's good practice to check in on the people around you, ask them how they are, and see if they need any help. I also keep the message threads on my phone so I can see whom I haven't checked on lately.

Our lives are based and built on relationships. The village itself is simply a collection of relationships. It's funny: I have been an active business owner for the past few years, and I made sure to build relationships by joining numerous organizations for female business owners. Recently I was part of a panel about women in business. As I sat on stage, it occurred to me that I was the only one on the panel who didn't have a master's in business administration. In fact, I never even took a business course in college. I studied theater.

When questioned about my credentials for giving tips to succeed in business, I explained why my theater degree was better than any business degree. Maybe I couldn't read a spreadsheet, but I knew how to read people, and I was able to hire the right people for my company to succeed. My company was a mini village, and I built the foundation of my company using the same concept I would use when creating any close community.

How Can You Become a Valuable Villager?

Let me start this section on becoming a valuable villager by talking about the word *values*. I use this word frequently, and I know I'll bring it up when discussing villages. Yes, I know the word tends to scare people because they immediately associate it with religion or morality. While values absolutely have a place within both, the word itself is defined differently for every person and every family. Right now, we are going to discover what it means to you. What do you value? There's no right or wrong way to answer this question. You might place a lot of value on attaining certain material goods, and I don't judge you for that at all. I have friends who place value on being great cooks, but I can't even boil water. No judgment here either.

When I was working with children, I saw how families placed values on different parts of their lives. Some valued education, and I ensured that the children paid close attention to their schoolwork. Others valued athletics, and it was the same deal, just a different value system. So why am I telling you all this? My first rule of thumb is "know thyself." Use the following exercise to figure out your value system before you join or create a community. Being self-aware is the first step to unleashing your value as a villager.

EXERCISE

Evaluating Your Values

Ask yourself the following three questions:

- *What does your ideal community look like?*

- *Why does your ideal community look this way? How do your values influence this village?*

- *How do you deal with someone whose values conflict with yours?*

These aren't easy questions to answer. I know, I had a hard time answering them myself. My values change as I move through different aspects of my life. However, I know that my true values are ones rooted in kindness, empathy, and compassion. I treasure these in myself and in others. I want every villager in my circle to have these core values. Something I should note: you might want to categorize the different values in your life and see how they influence your decisions. For example, what sort of values do you hold about wellness? They might be different than your values about finances. Finding how your values influence your life is an important step in understanding your actions. Many people don't realize their values guide their lives—they're everyday reflexes by the time we reach adulthood.

In short, to have a community of your own or to be an active member of someone else's village, it's important to communicate your needs and to understand the needs of others. Like the quiz you took earlier in the chapter, your goal in choosing relationships is to be seen, heard, and understood. I cast certain roles in my village, and I ask my villagers to assign roles for me. You might want to ask your friends and family what role you play in their world. As we move deeper into this book, we will study the six essential qualities that one should include when building a village. This will help you discover and nurture those qualities in yourself as well.

My first experience as a villager was when I was working with children. Back then, I was a hired villager. I had a certain set of duties I was contractually obligated to perform, but I was still part of their support system. But once I started nannying, I realized how many villages I was part of during the rest of my time. I thought back to when I was studying theater in college. Back then, I was in plays and was a valuable villager in that community. If you've ever been involved in a theatrical production, especially one with a limited budget, you understand how each person associated with the production is of intestimal worth. From the person who staffs the ticket booth to the director, each role is essential in making sure the show can go on. I performed in these types of productions and acquired the discipline one needs to be an actor. Memorizing lines was the first Herculean task, but it's not the focus of an actor's life. I didn't spend hours in class learning the art of memorization. My classes focused on exercises that helped me understand my emotions and learn how to draw upon my past experiences, so I could utilize them when I embodied a character on stage. When I was on stage, I wasn't Florence Ann Romano, I was the character the playwright created.

In retrospect, the exercises we had to do in acting class—the ones that made me travel deep within myself, pull out a variety of emotions, and study them—were a valuable tool for unearthing my inner villager. And taking the time to understand how a character thinks and behaves and differs from my own behaviors was another eye-opening experience that shaped the trajectory of my personal life and career.

So how do you become a valuable villager? I recommend first discovering what you value in yourself and others. Then reach out to someone who needs help and ask, "What can I do for you?" They might not be able to verbalize what they need, but the simple act of reaching out has already made you invaluable.

GUT CHECKS

- Make a list of the people you depend on.

- Make a list of people who depend on you.

- Are those lists equal? Why? Why not?

ACTION STEPS

- Donate items! This might sound easy, but the act of donating your stuff can help create an instant village as you help others in need.

- Be social on social media. For instance, if you notice someone posting about a lost job, a new baby, or a move to a new city, you can reach out to them.

- Be proactive and volunteer for needs in your community.

Can You Give Me Directions to This Village?

Creating a Village

The greatness of a community is most accurately measured by the compassionate actions of its members.
Coretta Scott King

Here's the truth: there are no pre-written directions to the village; you'll have to write them yourself. Most villagers don't just show up at your door. Instead, you must seek them out, and the prospect of assembling the group can often seem overwhelming. There are significant variables to consider, including who should be included, what the purpose of the community is, and, ultimately, whether it's truly working and living up to its fullest potential. This chapter cannot build a village for you, but it will guide you, step-by-step, through the process of assembling and maintaining a group of supportive friends and family you can rely on.

The first step is simply asking yourself, "What type of village do I need?" This sounds simple, but it's not. It's often difficult to admit our perceived shortcomings to ourselves and others. In identifying what communities we need, we should identify where we feel we are struggling and require help. Remember that in this "weakness," you will find strength. There is genuine courage in admitting that we need support, and it'd be best to keep this in mind as you engage in your soul-searching.

Self-discovery is not always comfortable, but it's necessary. The most fulfilling communities are inhabited by people who are conscious of their strengths and their limitations, and who know how to vocalize their need for support. Keep in mind that your soul-searching shouldn't stop once a village has been built; rather, you should continue to reflect on how you can best support, and be supported by, your fellow villagers.

I hit a low moment in my career when my digital content company was in economic distress. I was distraught; I felt immense responsibility for my employees, as they relied on me for their incomes. I didn't want to let them down, and I spent sleepless nights strategizing, attempting to save my business and their jobs. My identity was tied up in my career, and I was embarrassed to admit to anybody that I was struggling and desperately needed help. However, for the sake of my employees, I was forced to put my ego aside. I consulted with an entrepreneurial networking group. I admitted to them that I felt like I was drowning and that I needed somebody to come to my aid and advise me on what to do next. Though it was difficult to express this, the moment I did, I felt a flood of relief, as I no longer had to carry this burden alone.

The group shared the contact information of a business consultant, and I took the leap and reached out. Sitting in the subsequent meeting, I felt naked. Though frightening, it was also a much-needed instant gut check. The consultant asked me questions that had long lingered in the back of my mind and led to those sleepless nights. After confronting these issues, I worked through them and built a stronger company. I was fortunate enough to be able to sell my business while ensuring that all my employees would keep their jobs. I wondered what had taken me so long to reach out, when all I received once I did so was love and support. Fear held me back, as it does many of us. After overcoming toxic traits, I was able to embrace my new community. I realized that I wouldn't judge a young entrepreneur coming to me for advice, and thus I should not have expected that I'd be received with judgement.

As I noted earlier, there are no secret directions to a village. Still, there might be an entry fee. In my case, I hired a consulting team and used economic means to build a community. Of course, not all communities must be bought with money. In some cases, it can be as basic as bringing canned goods to a food drive or watching a neighbor's pet. That said, just because you pay to join a community

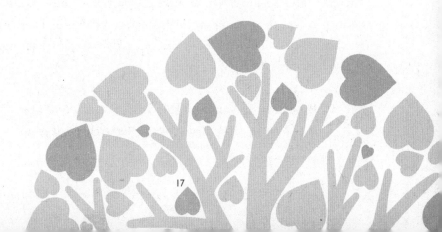

doesn't mean it's of greater or lesser value, or that your relationship with that community is somehow disingenuous.

Now, let's go chart our course to a village!

Drawing Up a Map to a Village

It's important to know the reason you want a village before you start figuring out the directions, so you can get yourself to the right place. It's kind of like planning a vacation: what you need determines where you go. For instance, if you want to take a week-long trip to recharge, you might spend it at a beach resort where you can sit under an umbrella sipping frozen beverages and watching the waves. If you are looking for adventure instead, you might visit another city or head for the wilderness. You know what you want from your trip. The same concept applies to the village. You should know why you need it before you create it. To answer this, look deep within yourself to see how you depend on others and how others depend on you.

Once you've identified a specific need, this is when you begin to assemble your village. And the fun begins! Sometimes this is rather straightforward—for instance, if you are new parent, joining a parents' group can provide you with support and friendship. If you're a college student looking for friends, joining a club or a sorority/ fraternity can be a great way to meet people. Sometimes, however, the map is less clear, and you might require guidance. There are five thought-provoking questions you can ask yourself to determine what village might be right for you.

1 **How long do you need this village?** Not all villages last forever, and that's okay. Remember all your

friends from college? Though you're probably not in touch with all of them now (at least not more than social media check-ins), they were valuable at the time. Some communities aren't meant to last forever. If you break your leg, you might need help while you recover, and reaching out to friends and family to build a makeshift recovery village might be vital. Once your leg heals, you won't need them in the same way anymore, but that doesn't diminish the important role they served, or the value of that specific village.

2 **How many villagers do you need?** You don't have to answer with a specific number, but it'd be good to have a sense of how large or small you want your community to be. Are you trying to connect with all the parents in your child's school to organize an event, or are you simply looking for a few close friends to support you through a difficult time? Setting these expectations early on will make it easier to create or join a group best tailored to your needs.

3 **How much time do you have to give?** Different villages require different contributions. After all, you only get as much from a community as you put in. Don't join a choir if you don't have the time to show up to rehearsal! That said, there are certainly creative ways in which you can serve as a villager. If you need somebody to drive your child to activities but cannot participate in a carpool yourself, perhaps you could provide snacks for all the kids. This is a thoughtful

and active way to thank the carpool parents, and one that could win you brownie points all around—no pun intended!

4 **How prevalent do you want this village to be in your life?** Are you looking for your primary community or a more casual group? If you're looking for something more serious, you might need to spend more time fostering your support system. But if you're looking for a group to help organize a fundraising event, building that village might be as simple as sending a foundational email.

5 **How can I remove myself from a village?** This might seem like a counterintuitive question—after all, this book is about building villages not disassembling them. However, it's important to acknowledge that your situation in life is subject to change, and a community that fits well for a while might be one that you later grow out of or simply want to take a hiatus from. Don't join (or stay in) a community in which you are asked to take on more than you can handle. And don't be afraid to admit that you can't handle it all when you feel overwhelmed. You should always be willing to communicate your boundaries, and sometimes that means taking a step back.

These five questions won't leave you with a tidy list of search results for your new village, but they are a valuable jumping-off point. I recommend taking time to pen a journal entry reflecting on these questions. You might realize that you are looking for a different community than you thought you were. A lot of this process is trial and error, so if you don't find the right fit immediately, that's fine. You can revisit these questions and then continue your search. Remember, the perfect village is waiting for you to help build it!

How Do I Know If My Village Is Working?

Once you build a village, you might wonder how to measure whether it is working. It's hard to measure satisfaction. It comes down to a gut feeling, something we often think we have but can't be quite sure. When I started college, I only knew a couple of people. I was anxious about building a community from scratch, and I worried that I wouldn't fit in. During my freshman year I joined Pi Beta Phi (my first choice!) and immediately found a sisterhood I could easily call my primary village. For my junior year, I took a leap of faith and studied abroad in England. It was an exciting and wonderful opportunity, but once in England I was brought back to those same freshman year worries. Although I traveled to England with a few students from the theater department, I didn't want to use that group as a crutch. I wanted to create new circles while studying abroad. A few hours into the program, I overheard a girl mention that she was a member of Pi Beta Phi. I nervously approached her and told her that we shared this sorority in common. After this, we became fast friends, and together we built a makeshift village of others in the program. My sorority was such a powerful community that it extended even beyond my campus chapter. In that moment,

I felt support, knowing I had a network of women around the world whom I could rely on. My sorority has helped me since then, providing me with valuable business contacts and lifelong friends, though it is no longer my primary village.

Of course, people don't always have the benefit of such structured institutions. As you get older, there are fewer built-in opportunities for relationship building, so you may have to put in the effort to create them. For example, people who work from home are more isolated than those who are surrounded by people in an office. Remote workers might have to work harder to create villages. We can create communities online—and believe me, I'm someone who is active on social media—but I know that virtual connection is no replacement for actual human contact.

The key to successfully working within a village is communication. Although people tend to talk a lot (I know I do!) it's often challenging to say hard things. If you're like me, you like to be polite. But even if you sugarcoat a comment, it still has the potential to upset someone. This might make you both momentarily uncomfortable, yet this risk is worth the reward. If you can't communicate how you feel, the village won't be able to serve you and the others in it. That said, we should be mindful of what we say and be able to explain our wants to the other members. You should definitely advocate for yourself, but I think we can all agree that to make the world a better place, we also need to help others.

Years ago, I was working with a family who valued education and were focused on their kids' grades. I noticed that their daughter was chronically overwhelmed by her parents' expectations. I knew I had to meet with her parents to explain what I was seeing. Filled with apprehension that I'd upset them and they'd believe I was blaming them, I decided to explain how the pressure was impacting their daughter's behavior. Fortunately, they were receptive and grateful for the insight into their daughter's struggles. While I was working with that family, I was part of their village, and I advocated for someone who couldn't do it for herself. How do you know if you should approach someone in your support system about something that you feel needs to be adjusted or, at the very least, discussed? I always say that if you feel something is awry, your feelings are valid. It's better to facilitate a discussion than to avoid the topic.

However, sometimes we can't recognize our own needs. We might be unaware that actions we think are helpful are actually harmful. There are times when we need someone else to do a gut check for us. I know this because it happened to me. I've wanted to be a mother my entire life, and when I reached thirty-five and was still childless and partnerless, I considered becoming a single mother by choice. Like everything in my life, I pursued it with great energy and immersed myself in the world of IVF. If you haven't done IVF, you might not know that this isn't an easy process. I fertilized some of my eggs with donor sperm and started the process to transfer an embryo. However, my body was exhausted and my levels were all over the place. I decided to press the pause button and give my body a break.

My network was made up of numerous cheerleaders who wanted to support me through this process, but I needed someone to ask me the hard questions, like "Are you sure it's a good idea to push yourself this hard?" The way I was pursuing results wasn't healthy, and my body was telling me I needed to rest. This meant I had to turn off the metaphorical timer I had placed in the corner, the one I used to put pressure on myself, and take a break. Obviously, this was when I needed my village. The cheerleaders let me know that this wasn't "the end" but "just a pause." When challenges occur, a lot of people live in a world of black and white; they don't see the gray. It took me a little while to adjust to this new time frame, but putting a hold on IVF didn't mean I couldn't become a mother. I had embryos there for whenever I wantd to use them. An insurance policy!

So how do you know if your village is working? If you feel over-whelmed by responsibilities, it's best to pause and address this. One way is to ask yourself if you feel comfortable communicating with all the members when it comes to challenging subjects. Occasionally you will need to reconfigure the village. Maybe a villager will take a break, or someone's role might change. Always remember that the village is constantly changing.

Something you should be mindful of when a village is functioning is that you shouldn't use it as a crutch. If you limit yourself to being with the people in a single village, you all might feel suffocated, and it could hinder your ability to grow. This means you should have check-ins with yourself and the other villagers and ask a couple of gut-check questions:

1   **How much am I relying on the village?** If you feel that you're relying on the village to meet *every* need, you might be overwhelming the other members.

2   **How much is the village relying on me?** If you feel that you're giving more than you're receiving, you need to speak to the other people in the group. You don't want to feel as if you are carrying everyone's burdens. The village is about reciprocity.

Once you've asked these two basic questions, you will uncover any flaws in the village and can address the issues thoughtfully.

Can I Create Multiple Villages?

You can, of course, create as many villages as you need, but be mindful of overextending yourself. You can have different circles for different aspects of your life. Examples include family villages, work villages, nonprofit villages, neighborhood villages, support villages (I've talked about these—we create them in times of crisis), and parenting villages. These communities enhance different parts of your life. Some of these might overlap, and some might sprout new villages. You might play different roles in each of these villages. Also, once you join a circle and perfect your skills as a villager there, you will find it easier to join others. The more people you meet, the more opportunities will come into your life.

As I said earlier, I joined an entrepreneur group when I launched my own business, and that led me to meet the consultants who helped me restructure my business model. If you find that you're either starting a new project or relocating, you might want to join a relevant group for that community. Most larger towns have groups on social media. People post everything from calls for volunteers to items they'd like to donate. Social networking platforms for communities are great launching points when trying to establish a village. Although I wouldn't say a digital platform is a complete village—it lacks the one-to-one component—these social networking communities help you engage with your "neighbors."

As you construct your villages, think about how each one serves a different purpose and how you plan to utilize and be part of that group. The first step is finding out what you'd like to offer the group. What skills do you think might work well in various groups? For example, perhaps you want to feel more involved with your local community. If this is the case, you might peruse social networks that focus on your neighborhood for activities you could be involved in. If your skills include nurturing plants, landscaping, or woodworking, you might find yourself connecting with people as you restore a community garden. The friendships you make as you're volunteering are a great way to establish yourself in your neighborhood.

A friend lamented that he couldn't find a good partner. He was trying to meet people in nightclubs, and it wasn't working. When we had a heart-to-heart, I explained that he should get involved with local organizations, where he could meet new people with varied interests. Yes, you can search for a partner online or at a local watering hole, but when you immerse yourself in a variety of communities, you make connections that can help you meet a person to date, find a new job, or find greater fulfillment in general. This is also how one searches for potential villagers. It's important to attract the kind of people you want to add to your life. This should be done with thought and care, as you cast people into various roles in your life.

That said, don't join a community expecting them to solve all your problems or to fix you. Although I talk a lot about villages, we have to work on ourselves before we can truly be part of one. (If you're struggling, of course, you could rely on one of your support villages to help you through a tough time.) My goal with this book is to get you to reflect on the relationships in your life and to see how you can elevate them through self-awareness. The gut-check questions are there for you to do the work on your own, and the action steps can be completed once you've addressed the gut-check questions.

Like me, you might participate in self-improvement rituals such as spring cleaning and digital detoxes, but what about taking a critical look at the roles of certain people in our lives? We don't usually take the time to do that when everything seems to be working; instead, our villages are recalibrated after a major life change or tough event. Remember how the world shut down in 2020? Millions of us lost the comforts of casual friendships. These are people you interact with every day, but they aren't the main players in your village. An article in *The Atlantic* stated that "peripheral connections tether us to the world at large; without them, people sink into the compounding sameness of closed networks."[1] This thought made me consider the structure of community, and the casual relationships we encounter each day without "village" consideration. Maybe you grab a coffee every morning before work and make small talk with the same barista. You might not have given this casual village a second thought until you lost them while staying at home.

We can work to become better members of a village, and once you figure out how you can help others, you'll see that others will help you in return. These various small communities create a gentle synergy that enhances everyone's lives.

GUT CHECKS

- Write about the time you feel someone helped you the most.

- Write about the time you feel you helped someone the most.

- How were those experiences different? Why?

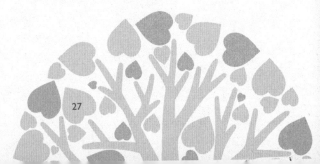

27

ACTION STEPS

- Make a list of your own needs and skills, and see where they overlap. For instance, if you need to feel that you're helping others in an essential way and you're a good cook, consider working in a shelter kitchen.

- Recognize something you need help with and reach out to one person to help you.

- Become an instant villager by simply checking in with a friend or family member and asking how they are doing.

How to Grow Your Village

The Various Villages You Can Inhabit

*In every community, there is work to be done.
In every nation, there are wounds to heal. In every heart,
there is the power to do it.*

Marianne Williamson

The beauty of learning to grow your village is that it's a central principle that can apply to all kinds of communities. Once you understand how to build one, and how to identify your villagers (remember the "Vetting for the Village" quiz in chapter 1?), you will start to recognize fully formed or even half-baked networks that are already established in your life. Perhaps the other parents at your child's school have formed a strong village, though you hadn't recognized it. Maybe your coworkers make up half of a village, and you feel that you can now build upon it and strengthen your relationships there. Although we all can be part of numerous groups, we can roughly divide our villages into two categories: primary and secondary.

When you think of your primary village, think of your besties or your family. These are the people closest to you, the ones you would call on in a crisis. Your secondary villages are equally as important but serve a different purpose. They help you in more specific ways: your coworkers, classmates, fellow parents, or members of a specialized support group. These might be more easily recognized, but that doesn't mean everybody you know is serving as a productive villager. Just because you know somebody from your gym class doesn't mean that they are a person who supports you, and for whom you provide support. Once you understand the notion of villagers, however, it will become a lot easier to build relationships that model this. That said, some people will not become part of your circle, instead remaining casual acquaintances, and this is all right. Though fostering relationships is important, don't strain yourself trying to force them.

To make it easier to identify the villages in your life, I've highlighted the two categories of villages, which can overlap:

- **Primary Village:** This one is your foundational community. It's made up of family, close friends, and other established relationships. This village will help you in all aspects of your life. You should tend to it often. In order to cultivate a mutually beneficial arrangement for all involved, you'll want to put in effort and be available to help the people in this village as much as they help you.

- **Secondary Villages:** These have specific goals. Although some of your primary villagers might fit into your secondary villages, the villagers in the secondary villages have clear-cut roles in your life. For instance, they might be coworkers, people you are collaborating with to create an event (think baby shower!), or those who are rallying to help someone who is sick. The secondary village might only exist for a predetermined length of time. Unlike your primary, the secondary village might have paid helpers, such as a nanny or a home health aide.

In the next six chapters, we will discuss the *six essential villagers* whom you need to form a complete village. These villagers are necessary for both primary and secondary villages. The qualities the villagers have are ones we will discover in ourselves and others. This will help us move past defining people generally as friends, relatives, or neighbors and get to know them on a deeper level. We will also see how you and the people in your life can help others in more specific ways. Each chapter includes exercises to nurture those aspects in yourself. Of course, there will be gut-check questions to keep you honest and action steps to help you make small moves forward in your life.

Before we delve farther into the two categories of villages, let's talk about finding potential villagers to populate your support systems. Although I'm quite social, I'm also a serious homebody and can spend all weekend hanging out by myself. Even if you're like me, which means being at home alone is your default setting, you would still benefit from having a village. In fact, being able to spend time by yourself shows that you enjoy your own company, and this is vital if you want to spend time with others. To be able to help others, you must first understand how to help yourself. This is a balancing act, and when you join a new community, you should pay attention to whether you are helping too much or too little. We will address the idea of *balance* throughout the book and talk about different ways you can check in with yourself once you form or join a village. But for now, we are going to embark on the journey of cultivating our first village.

Some of you might feel like you don't have a community. There are numerous reasons for this. When I moved to the West Coast, I missed the village I had built in Illinois. It's hard when everyone you love lives in another state. This happens quite often, though, and we must learn to establish ourselves in a new place. I notice that a lot of people who are in this situation seem to concentrate on the negative. I've had people tell me that they can't move somewhere because they don't have people there. I really get it, but I have a quick exercise to help you to discover potential friends and to create an instant village anywhere.

This two-part exercise applies to everyone—and I mean everyone. So, even if you've moved to another part of the world and don't know a soul, you can start building a support system this very instant. Okay, here's the exercise, and I promise it's an easy one.

Village Building

Part 1: The List

Make a quick list of all the people in your life who are there for you. Don't even think, just write the list. I know this sounds crazy, but they don't even have to be living. Write down everyone you've known and cared about. If you find this to be overwhelming, try scrolling through your contacts on your phone; doing so might make it easier.

After you've constructed this list, highlight the people who live closest to you. If you don't know anyone who lives near you, look at the people on the list and consider whether they have any friends you could reach out to who live nearby. The people on this list are your path to building a new village. Now, put that list aside and move to part two.

Part 2: The Questions

Answer these two questions:

- *Am I trying to create a primary or a secondary village?*

- *What can I offer the people in this village?*

If you moved, and you are literally starting from scratch in a new environment, you might want to create multiple secondary villages. Since you're still getting your bearings in a new place, you may want to recruit paid villagers, like a dog walker. You might want one parenting village and one work village. It's okay if the people in these villages overlap somewhat. You might even construct a group only to find that it doesn't work for you at all. If this happens, it's totally fine, because all communities are malleable. What you don't want to do is pick three people whom you have designated as your entire circle and have them serve in both your primary and secondary villages. That places heavy expectations on those people.

I always say that I discovered what a true village was when I was nannying, but in actuality it goes back a lot further. My brother Michael, who is not even two years younger than me, is autistic. When I was a young child, I watched my mother skillfully craft a village to help meet Mikey's needs. For example, when we'd go on vacation, my mother would ask my cousin to join us because she had a great relationship with Michael and gave him the attention he needed. Even today, Michael lives with my mother and cannot be left home alone. My mother still leans on her support system to care for him. She is never too proud to admit that she needs help. Growing up with people around me who helped Mikey was an early education on kindness and compassion. And I had to be his advocate, inspiring me to nurture caregiving qualities in myself and others. Over the years, numerous people have asked me about the challenges of having a brother like Michael, and I tell them it's a gift. I don't think I'd quite understand what compassion was if I hadn't grown up watching it in action. Lots of people say they care, but because of Michael, I know what active caring looks like at all stages of life.

I come from an old-school Italian family. My mom's parents lived with us for most of my life. My siblings and I had an indescribable bond with my Nana and Papa, and I was named after my Nana.

I always describe Nana as the love of my life and my best friend. Watching your grandparents age is a privilege, but it also comes with responsibility. Toward the end of Nana's life, when she broke her arm, she needed to wear an incontinence diaper. You have to understand that this was a super independent, modest woman, and now she was in a position of extreme vulnerability. She would only allow my mother and myself to help with changing her briefs. The first time I did this, Nana, looking down and shaking her head back and forth, said, "This is not how it's supposed to be. You should not have to do this for me."

And my response was, "You changed my diapers, and now it's an honor to do the same for you. It's the circle of life."

She smiled and said, "You're my angel. My little Florence Nightingale."

How Do You Utilize Your Village?

I can now talk endlessly about how I utilize my village, but when I wanted to hear how others used theirs, I reached out to my social media followers and asked them how they help their handpicked communities. How did they make it work for them? And what role did they play? My heart melted when responses flooded my inbox. The messages ranged from "help them feel seen" to "support whatever they are doing." People told stories of how they provided a shoulder to cry on, and others said they try to help by doing favors like watching their friends' kids. I was floored by the number of people who wanted to tell me how they help others.

Looking back through those responses, I want to highlight two response types that stood out. These were "allowing myself to be inconvenienced if it helps another" and "offering to help when they don't ask." These stuck with me because they are succinct instructions on how to care for another person. I want to tape these two statements to my wall to remind myself of these basic rules for being kind and helpful to others. Knowing when to offer help when someone doesn't ask for it isn't easy. This behavior, although rooted in kindness, can often feel intrusive and awkward, but sometimes a person isn't able to ask for help or feels guilty asking. This is when you could step outside your comfort zone and find a way to help a friend.

Speaking of helping fellow villagers, I received a considerable number of responses from people who were still looking for a village. Some responded that they wanted to help but didn't know how. Not knowing how to help someone is normal. In fact, simply questioning how we can help another person is a thoughtful act and should be commended. Doing this means we aren't just thinking about what we want to do but are thinking about what the other person needs. That said, we aren't mind readers, and we don't know what everyone wants or needs. The one aspect we can control is knowing what we can offer to others. Once you figure out what you can provide, you will be able to work within any community.

Years ago, someone gave my friend advice about how to balance being a single parent of school-aged children and having a career. They told her that despite being a working parent, she still might want to get involved in the school community in some way, even if it meant limiting herself to only one activity. My friend decided she would help with the book fair each year. Her children witnessed her working at the book fair, so they had consistent childhood memories of her at the school, and the PTA was grateful that she was eager to help at the annual event. I use this example because life isn't usually an "all or nothing" scenario. If you use your time wisely, you can balance various aspects of your life. Again, the key here is to avoid taking on too much.

This goes back to my original premise—if you know what you can offer others, you shouldn't have to guess what others want. Once you unleash your inner villager, people will take notice and see you display the characteristics of one (or possibly more) of the six essential roles—an *accepting person, a dependable person, a cheerleader, a communicator, a healer,* or *an organizer.* When you realize which villager(s) you are, you can open your heart and let love in! That said, if you find yourself with a role in someone's village and don't know how to help them navigate a difficult time, try reaching out to someone who has lived through a similar situation. For instance, I can rattle off a list of what someone might need if they're going through fertility treatments. In fact, I have written countless blog posts about this subject. You can also read articles or blogs about whatever issue they might be having in order to see how you can help them. I'm an avid researcher, and doing my homework on a subject empowers me. You don't have to do a lot, but make an active choice to find a way you can help them.

As we move through the book and discuss the six essential roles in more depth, you can begin to nurture certain traits within yourself. And once you start displaying these traits, you will no longer feel out of place in your community. My motto is (and will always be) "know thyself." It's not easy. I've done lots of work on myself, and I know how exhausting the process is. I'm not asking you to do a deep dive into yourself but to work to *find your language for caring.* Some people are great listeners. Others are reliable. We have myriad traits that can help us step into a role in someone's village; we need to be open to the idea of being part of a community.

Let's go back to the two-part exercise I asked you to do (page 33). You should have a list of names and answers to the two questions. Now think about the villages you want to create and start casting people into roles.

Who's in Your Primary Village?

You're still looking at that list of villagers, right? Since this is your primary village, you might have a mix of family and friends on your list. Right now, you're establishing the core circle that will help you through your everyday life. The people you choose to cast in this village are your besties, the ones you confide in, the ones you laugh with, the ones you've seen through bad times (and vice versa), and the people you want surrounding you at any milestone in life. Of course, this doesn't mean you don't have disagreements with these people or that everyone on your list is perfect (is anybody perfect?!), but these are people who know how to be real. Look at your list and find at least four people who fit into that your care circle. They don't all have to live nearby, but at least one of them should.

Another term I've heard used for this type of village is a *social support group*. While writing a blog post about the importance of a community in a new mama's life, I referenced an article that says, "Lack of social support can lead to isolation and loneliness."[1] In the introduction and in chapter 1, we discussed what studies have said about the impact loneliness has on your physical and mental well-being, and how prolonged loneliness could be fatal. Therefore, it's vital that you create this primary village. I can't see your list, but I'm sure there are people out there who feel like they don't even have a list. They might have written a bunch of names, but as they look at them, they start to cross each name off their list. Let me tell you, you're not alone. Countless of us feel that the people in their lives have failed them or that they have failed the people in their lives.

Let's start by recognizing there is no such thing as failing in life. Life isn't an algebra test (and let me tell you, I've failed a lot of those). No, life isn't about failing; it's all about moving forward while embracing uncertainty. Talk about a serious balancing act! This is why life is easier when you have a support system. When you look at that list and find that you don't really connect with anyone on it, please stop for a moment because I have a quick exercise for you. I know we haven't officially gone into detail about the six villagers you need in your group, but I'm going to list them again here:

- an accepting person

- a dependable person

- a cheerleader

- a communicator

- a healer

- an organizer

Soon we will delve into how these people play roles in our support systems. For now I'd like you to look at that list of roles and try to group your listed potential villagers by these traits. This means that someone you don't feel comfortable confiding in because they once told someone else a secret you didn't want to share might not get kicked off the list completely. Instead, we can see how that individual can work in other roles. Perhaps that person is one of the funniest people you know, and when you text them after a bad day, they will send a hilarious response. As the saying goes, laughter is the best medicine, and this means you can label that person as a "healer." Or maybe there is someone on your list who is a bit judgmental, and you'd avoid telling them anything personal because they would likely bring you down. Yet that same person has the skills, connections, and tenacity to get an event off the ground. You could label that person as an "organizer."

Take a few minutes and superficially label the people on your list. Don't stop and think about how they've wronged you or why they wouldn't be a good fit in your village. Try to focus on seeing if they display *any* qualities of the six roles. Once you're finished, I'm sure you'll see that the list isn't as short as you thought it would be.

Of course, we are trying to put together the primary village, so you will also have to include people you want to confide in and the people you want to be there for you. They don't all have to be "your person," but they should be people who make you feel comfortable and who have the capacity for caring. Earlier, I told you that your list could include people who had passed away. Of course, they can't really be *in* the village, but you might want to stop and focus on why you placed them on the list. What qualities did they have, and is there anyone on the list who displays similar qualities? Also, did the deceased person have anyone in their life you might reach out to? A good way to keep a dear one's memory alive is by connecting with people from their life. You might want to invite one their friends into your community. They, too, could likely benefit from support.

Once your list is complete, keep it close by. As we move through the book and learn about specific villager roles, you can refer to your list and see if friends or family members on it have other traits that might make them vital villagers in your primary village. So much of life is about finding the right people to be with you. I want to speak to all the single people out there: You don't have to feel alone because you haven't found "the one" to rely on. When you have a village, you have a network of people who help one another, and you don't need to rely on one person.

Recently I've been interviewed on TV about my decision to become a single mother by choice. Unfortunately, because of my thyroid issues, I paused this process. I bring this up because interviewers have asked if I have a boyfriend, and I don't.[2] I explain that my need to have a baby is stronger than my need to have a partner, but the reason behind that statement is that I don't have an urgent need to partner up—because I have a village. I've spent a lifetime establishing my primary village, and I've spent my adult life putting together numerous secondary villages that have nurtured me personally and professionally. I can't imagine believing that one person could fulfill all the numerous roles needed for their partner to be fully supported. I'm not saying being in a relationship isn't fulfilling. I want to fall in love and have someone to share my life with, but having a village will only strengthen that potential relationship.

Who's in Your Secondary Village?

The secondary village is easier to cast, because there's a specific goal or common theme to the group. As I mentioned before, it's okay to have an overlap between the two communities. Your best friend might be in the primary group and the parenting village. Or a sibling might also be cast in a secondary village. That said, you don't want your secondary village to be made up of mostly people who are in your primary group.

You have the names of your potential villagers, and you've answered the question on why you need one or multiple secondary groups. You might also want to determine how long you need these secondary villages for. An important thing to consider is how much time you can give to each secondary village. When creating a secondary support system, you should cast your role first. A secondary village is mutually beneficial, and to work properly, it'd be best if you set the tone. Let's say you're creating a parenting village. In my blog, I talk a lot about the need to have a parenting village, not only to help raise your child but also to help the parents. This means you might have one parenting village, but it satisfies multiple aspects of your parenting life. You have one friend who can teach your kids how to bake cookies, and another you can vent to after a rough parent-teacher conference. Meeting and establishing relationships with other parents fosters a community and lets you stay connected with your children as they grow.

We talked about the need to start secondary villages when we are in transitional periods in our lives. Many of these secondary circles are established during times of crisis, like when we need to support someone who is sick, or maybe we've moved to another city and need to find people who can help us navigate our new neighborhood. Starting over isn't easy; it's exhausting when everything is new. Recently when I left the city and moved to the suburbs, I felt blessed to meet the greatest neighbors anybody could ask for. These secondary villages have enhanced my life tremendously.

How did I start my secondary villages? The first one was accidental. Sometimes you can move to a new place and never meet your neighbors. There was at least a decade in Chicago when I didn't know anybody who lived in my large apartment building. Yet after I bought a place in the suburbs, I was instantly invited to a social gathering with my neighbors, and now we are part of one another's secondary village.

Established secondary villages aren't too hard to find. In fact, your children's school can be one. This doesn't mean you need to connect with everyone at the school, but it's a great place to find people you can identify with. This is also a moment when you stray from the names you have on your list and recruit new villagers. Since you don't know most of the people in an established secondary village, you should attend programs or events they're involved in and see how the people interact with one another. Armed with the list of traits and roles needed to complete a fully formed village, you'll be able to see where each member fits in. It's relatively easy to spot who is an organizer or a good communicator.

As you establish your village, think of the long- and short-term goals for this community. You might need your parenting village to help with carpooling, which is a logistical need that has a concrete timeframe, but you might also need the group to help you emotionally navigate the challenges at all stages of parenting. This is when you should seek out an accepting villager or a healer. Making sure you have a complete village is one way to ensure that the group can fully support you and the other villagers.

GUT CHECKS

- Why do you need a village?

- Do you think you've ever been part of one?

- What do you think you could offer a village?

ACTION STEPS

- Go digital. Choose something you love and create a group on social media or host an online event. If you don't want to create your own, join an online community for something you are passionate about.

- If a friend is planning an event, ask how you can help. Also, if there's a church group or local community group you're interested in, sign up to help with their events.

- Start small and be honest. Ask three people you know if they'd like to be part of your village.

The Accepting Villager

The Nonjudgmental One

To be fully seen by somebody, then, and to be loved anyhow—
this is a human offering that can border on miraculous.

Elizabeth Gilbert

On the night of my thirtieth birthday, despite celebrating with friends and family at a lovely rooftop party, I had the feeling I had failed myself. I had believed I'd be married and already a mother by thirty, but I wasn't. Yes, I was deeply loved and had my village celebrating my birthday alongside me, but something was missing. My mother tells people that as a young child, I loved playing with baby dolls and would often request that my mom take me to the hospital so I could have my baby (aka the toy store!). When I brought a new doll home, I immediately made it a birth certificate. So, it's no wonder my first career was nannying. However, as I got older and transitioned out of nannying, I realized I wanted to have a child. As I looked out at the lights of the Chicago skyline, I made a promise to myself that if I wasn't married by thirty-five, I would have a baby on my own.

Flash forward five years. I know more about my follicle count and estrogen levels than I ever expected. When I started writing this book, I was chronicling my journey through IVF on social media. I loved sharing my experiences with my village because it helped me feel connected to others who are going through or contemplating this process. When I first started IVF, there was nobody to talk to. None of my friends had experience with fertility treatments. When I connected with women online who were undergoing treatment, I felt like I had stumbled upon a secret IVF club.

Yet, before I completed my two egg retrivals, I opened my messages and found one from an acquaintance who had been following my journey on social media. Her message, unwarranted and unwanted, questioned the decision I was making to maybe become a single mother by choice. I sent her a polite yet curt reply, but she didn't take the hint. She continually sent me articles on the impact of raising a child without a father. I asked her, "Don't I have enough love for the baby?" She stood by her belief that my child shouldn't be raised without a father. After countless messages, perhaps because she couldn't change my mind about raising a child on my own, she decided that I should adopt, rationalizing that there were great numbers of children in need of a home, and this would be a better path for me.

I was shocked. She had no right to judge my decision. I was upset, but also knew that I wasn't alone. As I mentioned, I found my IVF village on social media. Many of the women following me there were undergoing IVF and becoming single mothers by choice, and I bet they faced similar reactions. I reached out to my social media village and made a short video discussing this woman's messages. I received many comments from followers who sympathized with me.

A few weeks later I received another message. Maybe the impassioned messenger watched my video, or maybe someone else helped her understand how hurtful her messages were. She apologized. I was shocked. She reflected on her previous comments and realized it wasn't her right to judge my choice. I thanked her for that message. I understood that when she sent the previous messages, this woman had thought she was being helpful, although that couldn't have been further from the truth.

When dealing with this experience, I thought about what my Nana always said to me: "At some point you have to accept people for who they are, not for who you want them to be." I try to live by this motto, but it isn't always easy. It's hard work to accept someone for who they are. If you don't believe me, look at the unfortunate number of families and friendships that shatter when people have opposing political views. We must work to accept people, but we must learn to accept ourselves first. This is the reason I'm starting with the accepting villager—because acceptance is at the foundation of every support system. But how do we learn to be accepting? It's a skill that takes practice.

What Does the Accepting Villager Look Like?

We'd like to think that everyone has good intentions, or at least that the people we choose to have in our lives are looking out for our best interests. I truly believe the woman who messaged me had good intentions and wanted to stop me from making what she thought was a choice that would negatively impact my potential unborn child's future. Plenty of folks believe they are well-intentioned, yet they aren't self-aware enough to understand someone else's needs. The accepting villager can navigate other perspectives and beliefs in a nonjudgmental manner. They don't assume they know how you feel or what you're thinking.

I'm sure you think that you're accepting, but I have a quick exercise for you. This is another instance where you might want to take out a journal and jot down an entry.

EXERCISE

Accepting

Answer these two questions:

- *When was the last time someone revealed a problem or secret to you?*

- *What was your initial reaction to what they revealed?*

There are no correct answers to these questions. This is an exercise for you to pause and reflect on how you reacted to a situation. You can also reverse the question and ask yourself about the last time you revealed something to a friend and how they reacted. Did they really hear you? Did you feel seen? Or did you feel judged?

Think about how their reaction impacted you. If you felt they were truly accepting, what made you feel that way? If you felt heard and seen, try to figure out what that person did to make you feel that way. And then try to replicate that behavior the next time someone reaches out to you with a problem. But maybe you didn't feel heard or seen. Or maybe when someone was divulging something to you, you couldn't help but judge them. You might have certain values that you feel strongly about, but to be accepting, you mustn't impose your value system on another person.

This reminds me of a young couple featured on my web series, the parents of a one-year-old and a three-year-old.[1] They were fortunate to have loving and dependable grandparents in their village, who picked their children up from daycare. The couple reached out to the web series because they were upset that the grandparents were giving their children too many sweets and letting them play with balloons, both of which worried the parents, and they wanted to talk about cutting out the sweets and the balloons without making the grandparents feel bad for their actions. I listened to their problems, and then I showed them a chart I had created to help deflate confrontational behavior. I was inspired to make it while employed as a nanny, as it helped me discuss issues with the families I worked for. Since then, I've used it frequently in my personal and business life. I am a strong believer that we should look inside ourselves before we complain about another's actions.

This chart starts with the basic question "Is this unsafe?" If the parents answered yes to this question (as these parents did regarding balloons), I advised them to find a time to sit down and address the matter. If the answer was no, the next question to consider is whether the behavior goes against their family values.[2]

I've spoken about values before, so you know I maintain that differing values must be addressed but also accepted. When I was a nanny, each family I worked for had their own set of values, and I had to accept that and work within them. This family didn't want the grandparents to give their children sugary treats every day. Depending on how many sugary treats the kids are getting, it *could* be a health and safety issue—but in this case, the parents concluded that it was not unsafe. Therefore, these parents had some work to do. They had to stop sweating the small stuff and accept other people's value systems even if they disagreed with them.

Just because you accept someone else's values doesn't mean you have to change your own. If you can accept other points of view, you'll be rewarded with a rich variety of people in your village. Not everyone has to have the same beliefs, but everyone can try harder to be more accepting.

The woman who messaged me about IVF and the grandparents from the web series ultimately had to accept the needs of the person they wanted to help. An accepting villager thinks about other people but doesn't project their thoughts onto them. A friend was telling me about her good friend Carolyn, whose village she was part of when Carolyn was undergoing cancer treatment. Carolyn expressed to her that everyone assumed she was miserable due to her diagnosis. One person even said, "You are living my worst nightmare." We all have ideas of how someone is feeling when they are going through a tough time, but we might not be correct. Carolyn was battling a potentially deadly disease, but she also laughed every day and had precious good days. She was upset that people assumed how she was feeling. Yes, she struggled and did need help as she underwent chemotherapy, surgery, and other treatments, but she didn't want assumptions and pity.

We can empathize with someone, but we can't know what they're feeling unless they tell us. The accepting villager is often the person you can be honest with, and they embrace that honesty without judgment. Again, being an accepting person isn't an easy task. I'm sure you're imperfect like me—like most of us—and you catch yourself being judgmental. I recall when a good friend got a tattoo and I wondered why she didn't choose a more discrete part of her body for the image she had chosen. Why did the entire world need to see this? Was this the image of herself that she wanted to portray to strangers? Then I stopped myself and realized that she wanted this tattoo and I had to respect it. She didn't ask me to get a matching tattoo. This wasn't my body, so why was I being so judgmental?

What Role Does the Accepting Villager Play?

The accepting villager should be the first person (role) you cast for your village. If you are going through a tough time, they will be the person you initially reach out to, because they are an active listener. They will acknowledge your problem, which is the first step in helping you move forward with your life. This is a person you probably already know and can locate easily. Think about someone you've revealed a secret to, the one friend you know will still be there after the revelation. They won't ask you to do any penance or recite prayers for forgiveness. They will accept you despite the confession and continue to see you as yourself. They won't brand you with a scarlet letter or tell other people what you divulged. They will keep it to themself because they understand that confessions are part of having a deep relationship.

I love the show *Grey's Anatomy*, and I recall in one of the early seasons, one of the main characters, Cristina Yang, described her best friend, Meredith Grey, by saying, "She's my person. . . . If I murdered someone, she's the person I'd call to help me drag the corpse across the living room floor. . . . She's my *person*."[3] I instantly thought of my best friend when I heard that speech. Of course, I wouldn't want to make my best friend an accessory to murder, but we get that the quote wasn't about murder at all. The quote was about someone who could walk into your life and help you, no matter the situation, without any judgment.

I should note that the accepting villager doesn't have to be your best friend. It could be a neighbor, a coworker, or someone you've met in other areas of your life, but it ought to be someone who will be by your side no matter what you say. When I decided to make my initial call to the fertility clinic to see what my options were for possibly becoming a single mom by choice, the first person I told was my mother. She is my essential accepting villager. When I told her what I was going to do, she listened and said she'd love to accompany me to the appointment. I'm sure this wasn't the way she wanted me to tell her I was having her grandchild. I'm also sure that despite not pressuring me or saying anything overt, she wanted to see me married and having a baby with a partner, and not having to do this on my own. Yet she backed my decision and didn't say anything to me that wasn't 100 percent supportive. As we drove to the clinic for this first meeting, I was nervous and wasn't sure if I was making the right decision. I admitted this to my mom, who reassured me that she had raised me with the help of her mother, and she would do the same for me and my child. This made me feel as if I was upholding a family tradition and helped me realize that if it was meant to be, I could do it.

As you can see, the accepting villager helped me move forward, and I believe that's the essence of this role. In order to create the rest of your village, it's important to accept the situation at hand and have someone there by your side. The power of acceptance is enormous, and acknowledging someone's pain without trying to solve their problems is one of the greatest gifts one human can give another. When someone is experiencing trauma, saying something well-meaning to them, such as "It will get better," might seem like the right statement to make but it's more powerful to accept that their intense feelings are natural and it's okay to feel them. There is no timeline for getting better. Due to our discomfort surrounding tough emotions, we often tell people a range of platitudes to show that we care, but simply acknowledging their circumstances and standing by them can help them grow stronger.

Now let me be clear: acceptance doesn't only need to take place in tragic or earth-shattering circumstances. Here's an example: when a bunch of my girlfriends were getting married, I accepted their news and was thrilled for them though I yearned to find someone I wanted to share my life with. The act of putting our emotions aside so we can help or rejoice alongside another person is the key element of an accepting villager.

The accepting villager doesn't have to live near you and can be anyone who will help you through a transitional period without judgment. Recently one of my friends told me she was moving to Texas. This gal is a true Midwesterner and has braved enough Chicago winters to deserve to live in a more temperate climate, but I was utterly heartbroken. I had spent the last few years helping her by babysitting her two kids, and now I was about to possibly embark on my motherhood journey. My response to her was, "How rude! I helped you all this time, and now you're abandoning me?"

I'm totally kidding about saying that. I don't need her to babysit, but I am going to miss her a lot. She's been part of my life for what seems like forever. She called me and was upset about relocating and establishing herself in a new community. There was fear in her voice when she asked, "How am I going to do it?" I quoted the show *Sex and the City*, when Carrie Bradshaw is afraid to move to Paris and Samantha Jones reassures her, "Believe me, your fabulousness will translate."[4]

I thought about how I met my friend. We were in college. I only knew two people going to my college. I spent the summer before college both excited and terrified (yes, this is possible!). When I got there, I was fortunate to meet a group of girlfriends who were ultimately as valuable (maybe more so) as my diploma. New people were going to come into my friend's life—she just hadn't met them yet. And once she did, I knew she would wonder how she had ever gotten by without them, which is exactly how I felt when I graduated from college.

But back to the present. I wanted to scream, "DON'T MOVE," but I didn't. I thought about the village and tried to play the role of accepting villager. Even though I'd miss her terribly, I accepted she was leaving. I knew this was the best move for her family. I told her that I'd forever be part of her support system, but I added that between the families she would meet at her children's schools and in her town, she'd find a community. But how would she find her accepting villager? Yes, I could still be that villager to her, despite the geographic limitations, but she can have more than one. If she wanted to find one nearby, how could she find one? What would they look like?

The accepting villager isn't difficult to find, even if you're new to a place. They are usually a person who has solid friendships, and you can recognize them by watching how they interact with others. To be accepting to others, you must first accept yourself. This means the accepting friend might be open about challenges they've experienced. My mother was my accepting villager when I told her about my goals with IVF. But I've had other accepting villagers in different stages of my life.

When I graduated from college and moved to Los Angeles, leaving my grandparents was the hardest part. When I moved, I told them I could see the heartbreak on their faces, but Nana said, "I don't have to like it; I love you enough to let you go." I appreciated this comment tremendously, although she confessed years later that she had prayed nightly for my return, which might be why I lasted in Los Angeles a mere eighteen months. All joking aside, she accepted my decision to completely change my life, and she did so without judgement or question.

Your accepting villager should support you the way my grandmother supported me. But despite the name, they should not provide *unconditional* acceptance. A good accepting villager doesn't enable destructive behavior; they say something when a decision seems dangerous or objectively wrong.

When I divulge something to a friend, they often want to help solve the problem at hand. But the accepting villager isn't there to fix your issues or make them go away; they are there to acknowledge them without judgement (unless they feel what you're doing isn't safe). Support is different than problem solving, and you need someone who lets you unload your issues without believing they know what's best.

How Can I Be an Accepting Villager?

The first step in becoming an accepting villager is to question yourself and the way you interact with others. Are you meeting friends and family members where they are and not where you want them to be? If not, why not? I know it's hard to see things from another point of view, but that is essential when unleashing your inner accepting villager.

One friend of mine, a creative writing teacher, told me that her favorite writing prompt is asking her students to set a story in a place they've never been. She tells her students to think about where they gathered the information to create an environment they've never experienced. Was it from TV, books, magazines? The same idea applies to people. If a friend is going through a divorce, maybe you haven't been through one yourself (or even if you have, we each have different experiences), you can only imagine what they are feeling. Ask yourself, where did you cultivate your perception of how it feels to be this person going through a divorce? If you think you know what they're feeling based on experiences in your personal life, please put those experiences aside. If you've never experienced anything like what they're going through, put all your preconceived ideas away and *listen to their story*. Not one story is the same, and you should hear your friend's story as their own. Now is the time to acknowledge their voice. You have the chance to be Meredith Grey to their Cristina Yang and help them drag the body across the living room without asking any questions. You can be their person. The accepting villager is someone's person, and that is a gift. We spend so much time cluttering our lives with superficial relationships. Getting to know and accept a person for who they are benefits both you and your friendship.

When I was a nanny, I had to earn the trust of each family who employed me. My job was to develop relationships with the family members, which enabled me to play multiple roles within their community. Every family has their own way of parenting. Some parents are hyper-focused on structure and achievement, and others are more laid back about letting their children explore. My job wasn't to judge these families but to watch their children.

I have long said that I modeled my career after the film *Mary Poppins*; I loved the lessons about family one learns from watching it. I should mention that while I would classify Mary Poppins as an accepting villager, like many of us she also embodies qualities of the other roles. At the moment, we are going to focus on her role as an accepting villager. For those of you who aren't familiar with the film starring Julie Andrews, it's about a magical nanny. The children write their own advertisement for the perfect nanny, and then a great wind blows away all the traditional nannies lined up to interview for the job posted by their father (he had ripped up the children's advertisement, but the children were unaware of this fact). Mary Poppins flies in on an umbrella and brings fun into these two children's rigid lives. Along with her friend the chimney sweep, she teaches the parents to appreciate their children and to make time for them.

She accepted Jane and Michael Banks, her charges, for who they were: young children in need of attention. Although she did fly in on both an umbrella and an inflated ego—from her carpet bag she pulled out a tape measure that she proudly announced had sized her up as being "practically perfect in every way"[5]—she also formed a deep relationship with the family by observing them. Mary Poppins had confidence, and that's a vital quality for an accepting villager. This is my observation and not hard science, so you might not agree, but I find that someone who is confident with their life choices is often less judgmental and more accepting of others.

An accepting villager should be observant. Watch what a friend is doing, and accept it. If their behavior is harmful, address it in a non-judgmental manner. This is often the tricky part, but the key is to think about what is best for that person, not what you think is best. This might sound confusing, but it's just practicing the act of offering support and not an opinion.

GUT CHECKS

- Would you consider yourself an accepting villager? Why?

- Have your values ever clashed with someone else's values? How did you react?

- Name a time you were accepting of another person or a situation.

ACTION STEPS

- When a friend tells you about a problem, listen without judgement. Don't try to solve it. Instead, acknowledge it. The accepting villager gives a person the space to articulate their needs.

- Before you judge, ask yourself if what someone is saying or doing is unsafe. If it isn't, accept their values and understand that they may not match your own but work to address the issue of safety.

- Acknowledge that you can't know what someone is thinking. Instead, ask what they need.

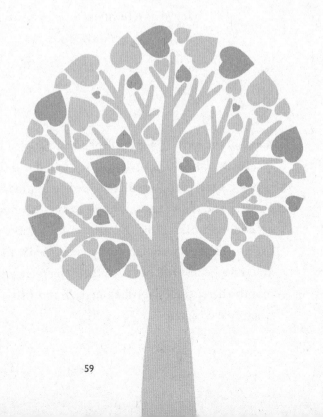

The Dependable Villager

The One to Contact in an Emergency

Try to be a rainbow in someone's cloud.

Maya Angelou

Some of the most fiercely independent people I know paused when I casually asked them whom they put down as their emergency contact. One friend even confessed that when she moved to this country and didn't know a single person, she made up a name and an address while filling out a form for a job that required her to list an emergency contact. Of course, that's an extreme example, and most people will not need their emergency contact. After a few months here, she established herself and had a few names to list when I asked again.

The dependable villager doesn't have to be your emergency contact, but your emergency contact has to be dependable. We're going to focus on how you can find a dependable villager and utilize that person in your world. We will also discuss how you can nurture these traits in yourself.

But first, let's start out with a hard truth. We all have flaws. That doesn't mean we aren't dependable, but we must be aware of our flaws and make sure they don't get in the way of helping another person. For instance, maybe you are frequently late but are otherwise dependable. This means you shouldn't write yourself off—you are more than the chronically tardy friend—but you might not want to be the person who gives someone a ride to a job interview.

The dependable villager takes various shapes in your life, and there are varying degrees of dependability. I have a good friend who habitually overextends herself. She has the best of intentions, but because she wants to help everyone, she winds up being a bit unreliable. She's the first person I might call when I'm in trouble, but she might not be available to help in big ways. We may well have people in our lives who are more than happy to help in small but dependable ways. Think about the last time someone offered to run an errand for you or helped you shovel your driveway. These people are of equal importance as the accepting villager when you're cultivating a village.

Let's return to the emergency contact. After I spoke to the friend who had created a fictional emergency contact, I began to think about my emergency contacts. This is one of those moments of truth that helps us realize what roles people play in our lives. Fortunately, I come from a large family and have a close relationship with my mother, who happens to live nearby. However, there were times when I was living on the West Coast and abroad when I didn't have my family nearby. At that time, being asked a basic question like "Who is your emergency contact?" made me feel exposed and vulnerable. I felt alone, and I'm someone who loves to have people in my orbit. On the flip side, it also motivated me to find people and build new communities. To succeed in a new environment, we can't spend our time worrying about who isn't in our lives. We need to seek out people we do want in our lives. The first step is taking small, dependable actions for others in your world.

How do we find dependable people we want to bring into our lives? Also, if we do find them, should we put them down as an emergency contact? According to a comprehensive online legal guide, "The ideal emergency contact is able to talk to medical professionals about medical history, allergies, chronic conditions, and current medications. In some cases, they even make medical decisions for their loved one. This can be life-saving in an emergency, so it's important to choose someone who is willing to do the job, can answer those questions, and who also has the legal right to act on your behalf."[1] If you're living far from home, it should be someone who has access to significant people in your life so they can contact others. Although the emergency contact will most likely not be called upon to act, this is a big responsibility. You should not put someone's name down unless they are aware of it. Also, you want to choose someone who is geographically close to you. You might have the best friends and family in the world, and even though they will hop on the first flight out to be with you, they shouldn't be the first names you put on an emergency contact list.

The reason people might panic when they fill in this empty space on a form is because there is a lot of weight surrounding this. Nobody wants to imagine a worst-case scenario or to picture their friend standing beside them making medical decisions on their behalf. No, we want to enjoy the people in our lives and have a nice dinner or go to a concert with them. Obviously you can do both, but the dependable villager is someone you can rely on to assume more burdensome tasks.

When we imagine facing a crisis, we take stock of our relationships. Who would we turn to if we got sick? We'll discuss how to cultivate this sort of relationship so that we have those people to rely on. But they are often already in our lives.

What Does the Dependable Villager Look Like?

From an emergency contact on your waiver when you go skydiving to the neighbor who waters your plants when you're out of town, there are any number of ways you rely on dependable villagers. The dependable villager isn't usually just one person, but your *central* dependable villager should be someone who lives less than thirty minutes away and can spare small intervals of time. The key factor to consider when selecting a dependable friend or family member is proximity. I don't mean this in the physical sense, though that is an important factor, but also in an emotional sense. Not only should your dependable villager be close enough to you that they can support you day-to-day, but you should be comfortable enough with them to be willing to ask for help. There isn't any point in having a dependable villager if you don't feel that you can ask them for favors without shame or embarrassment. Don't assume that a person can serve as your dependable villager; have an open and honest discussion with whomever you choose, so that you can draw boundaries together. You don't want to take advantage of somebody's kindness, nor do you want to ask more of somebody than they can give. If possible, try to be your dependable villager's dependable villager in turn. This reciprocity might make you feel more comfortable asking for favors and alleviate any guilt you might feel. This two-way street isn't always possible, but there are certainly other ways to show appreciation.

This two-question proximity exercise is a quick way for you to determine whether you've found a central dependable villager.

EXERCISE

Dependable Villager Proximity

Please take a few minutes to answer the questions below:

- *What is your physical proximity to this person?*

- *What is your emotional proximity to this person?*

If you are on the hunt for a dependable villager in your life, brainstorm people who are ideal to cast for this role. You might have more than one person, and that's okay. Once you've found an appropriate candidate, reach out and have a conversation about the possibility of becoming each other's central dependable villager. Be sure to have an open and honest discussion about their boundaries, and see if they agree that you're emotionally connected enough to rely on each other.

Types of Dependable Villagers

Now that you've found your central dependable villager, you'll want to populate your village with other dependable people—but which ones do you need? Here's a quick roundup of dependable villagers you'll consistently see in various communities. I bet a few of these are familiar to you.

The Emotionally Dependable Villager
This could be your central dependable villager, or perhaps someone who is there only for your emotional needs. This dependable villager need not be in close physical proximity. They might double as your accepting villager.

The Casually Dependable Villager
This might be a neighbor who keeps a copy of your key in case you get locked out or does other small but vital tasks.

The Physically Dependable Villager
Sometimes you need someone to help move your couch, or maybe your friend has a toolkit or a good shovel.

The Reliably Dependable Villager
This is the person you might ask to join your carpool or help you with other time-sensitive activities.

You can have more than four dependable villagers, but you might also have fewer. In fact, a couple of people can serve multiple roles. The dependable villager is essential when you're creating a secondary village to take care of someone like an elderly parent, a sick friend, or a child. If you've ever been a caregiver, you know how tax-ing it is. According to Caregiver.com, "approximately 43.5 million caregivers have provided unpaid care to an adult or child in the last twelve months."[2] In fact, people at my stage of life are referred to as the "sandwich generation" because so many of us must take care of our children and our aging parents simultaneously.

If you are a caregiver, you shouldn't take on the task alone. This is when you most need a support system. You can create a secondary village to help you care for this person. I mean, wasn't the phrase "It takes a village" popularized because it highlights the value of com-munity? Before I even decided to pursue becoming a single mother by choice, I cast all the people in my support system in roles that would help me raise my child. Of course, that's a joyous occasion. It's less pleasant to think about who you'll need if (God forbid) you get in an accident, but it's good to have a solid group of people you can rely on if that happens. The dependable villagers are the ones who tend to populate care villages.

When a friend was going through cancer treatments, an organizer villager in her life recruited various dependable villagers to sit with her during chemo, deliver meals to her home, and check on her throughout the day. The casually dependable villager in that scenario could have sim-ply cooked a meal and dropped it off. There doesn't need to be an ongoing commitment—even small gestures of comfort and support can be enough, espe-cially if more than one person contributes in some way.

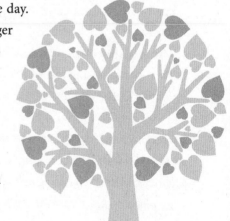

What Role Does the Dependable Villager Play?

I started with the most vital of all dependable people in your life—the emergency contact—but it gets easier from there, I promise. I started with such a dire example to establish the importance of the dependable villager. Hopefully the idea of finding an emergency contact didn't create anxiety for you. From now on we'll talk about people who fill dependable roles, but ones not as "life or death" as an emergency contact. What role the dependable villager plays in your life depends on the circumstances. Let's say you are trying to plan a rummage sale for a local charity. It wouldn't work if you didn't have dependable volunteers who signed up to collect donations, post signs, and work the event.

People who volunteer often make dependable villagers. People who can find the time to help others and stand by their commitments usually understand the importance of other people. When you look outside yourself and see how you can help others, you might ignite dependable qualities within yourself. Remember though, that just because you can't spend extensive time on charity work doesn't mean you aren't dependable in other ways. Sometimes our personal commitments are overwhelming and we can't be there for people. What we want to do and what we can do are not always perfectly aligned.

In the past few months, I've seen my world change. During this time I've gone through two egg retrievals, wound up in the ER with kidney stones, and decided to pause my IVF—so I'm not sure how dependable I've been. There are days when I can barely hold it together. Trying to work, manage my health, and write this book is enough to unintentionally distance me from the people I care about. During these times you see the people who are there for you. My friends and family have rallied for me, driven me to doctors' appointments, and stood by me. The dependable woman everyone knows as Auntie Lo has been on hiatus, and I couldn't be there for everyone in the way I'd like to be. The first step to being dependable is acknowledging how much you can do, and at this point, I can only help out in small ways. For instance, I do not leave texts unanswered, and I make time to chat with friends who need to talk. These might appear to be little acts, but letting someone know you are there, and being honest with them, is a lot harder than it appears.

While I was dealing with these medical issues, I thought about an interview I did on Instagram. A couple of months ago, I interviewed parenting coach Tia Slightham about positive discipline, but like many of my conversations it veered toward the topic of villages. She said that when she moved to a place where she didn't know anyone, she, too, had to construct a new village. When she arrived in her new city, she found herself spending her days alone with a four-month-old while her husband was at work. As an educator who yearned to teach, this situation proved untenable. Since she didn't know a single person besides her husband, she needed help. In the interview she stressed that asking for help isn't a weakness but a strength. Once you understand how to ask for help, you become stronger. Tia looked for outside (paid) villagers to assist her, after which she had more opportunities to pursue her career. She now had more room to *breathe.* Tia was quite passionate when she said we shouldn't feel guilty abut wanting or needing to pay someone to come to our aid.[3]

This means that sometimes we're required to hire a dependable villager. For years, I was the hired dependable one, the one who showed up every day and watched someone's children. Slowly I became an established fixture in their lives. Your relationships with hired dependable villagers aren't strictly transactional; you can have an established personal relationship with them. I'm still in contact with every family I nannied for, and I have attended weddings and other celebrations for those families. There is no shame in hiring extra help. That said, sometimes we don't have the economic means to do so. This is becoming a crisis in the United States. Just this morning I read an article in the *New York Times* entitled, "Who Will Take Care of America's Caregivers?" which discussed how people who are hired to help elderly or sick people are often grossly underpaid, and family members who serve as unpaid caregivers are exhausted. What stood out to me in this op-ed was this sentence: "This is not a uniquely American challenge. Japan, with the world's oldest population, has a term for the stress and exhaustion of family caregivers: *kaigo jigoku*, or 'caregiving hell.'"[4]

You may have picked up this book because you can no longer care for someone on your own. I recall the many nights I spent at my grandparents' bedside when my nana had a broken hip and after multiple other hospital visits. My grandparents were fortunate to have a large family, so we had a built-in family village with several dependable villagers, but not all families are as fortunate. Even with a large family, the toll of taking care of grandparents is often overwhelming. This is why it's vital that we find dependable villagers in our lives. Yes, sometimes we must pay them for their constant dependability, but other times we can find volunteers who don't mind helping and would even value being a part of our communities.

How Can I Be a Dependable Villager?

Before we can become someone's dependable villager, it's crucial that we understand our limitations. Although you might have the best intentions, you can't take on this role if you aren't able to fulfill the responsibilities that come with it. As I mentioned before, I am currently going through a challenging time, and I can't do a lot to help others. Yet I learned what great kindness people have and how they feel truly satisfied when they see they've helped me. In watching my village care for me, I've gained a deeper understanding of how to become more dependable. Often, we think we're dependable because we show up for someone, but it goes beyond that.

I was in the ER recently for my kidney stones. After months of medical procedures, you'd think I'd be a pro at this, but that is not the case. Especially when I couldn't even have my dependable villager at my side because of COVID-19 regulations. Sometimes we are in situations when our person can't be with us. Despite folks lamenting the negative impact of social media, there are times when I feel solace from connecting with my digital village. I posted from the ER and within minutes I had a flurry of texts from various dependable villagers in my life asking, "How can I help you?"

How can I help you? is a question we all ask in times of trouble and when we want to do something for a person we care about. Yet this isn't an easy question to answer. While I attempted to sit up in a hospital bed, wearing an N95 mask and hooked up to an IV, this question stumped me. Although I knew I needed help, I wasn't sure how to answer that question. This was a learning moment and a teaching moment, during which I learned how to ask for help but also observed how dependable villagers approached this invitation to my care village.

Some invitees knew what to do because they had been there before. Hearing stories of others dealing with chronic kidney stones made me feel less alone. Reading their tips for dealing with this issue helped me figure out a personal care plan for myself. In this instant village, I had to call upon my central dependable villager, but there were also other dependable people who offered to drop off a meal, drive me to follow-up appointments, and so on. I didn't ask these casually dependable villagers for help; they volunteered. This is the important lesson I learned from this experience. People don't always have to be invited to a village; they can invite themselves. They didn't ask me to identify what I needed; they offered a specific service they knew I would need. From kind words to an offer to drive me to the pharmacy, they were there for me in both large and small ways. Now I know it can be valuable to offer concrete assistance rather than simply asking, "How can I help you?"

So how can I reciprocate when I'm back on my feet? Well, first I have to understand what I can offer someone. I'm the worst cook in the world, and nobody would want to eat anything I've prepared, so I'm not going to be someone's casually dependable chef. But I can babysit my friends kids, volunteer to carpool, or even spend time with someone who needs some extra TLC.

The way you can be dependable is by reaching out and offering to help someone. Don't wait for an invitation—invite yourself. Jot down a list of ways you can help someone. When my friend was widowed and trying to keep her family afloat, one of her friends who was also a teacher offered to help her children do their homework. This was a weekly meeting where the friend went over the assignments and helped the children keep up with their work during a time of intense grief. Be inventive and figure out how you can help someone. It can be as easy as picking up something from the store or visiting with them. Once you get into the practice of helping others, you will show others you're reliable.

GUT CHECKS

- Who would you list as an emergency contact?

- Who would list you as an emergency contact?

- Is that the same person? Why?

ACTION STEPS

- Offer up your services! What can you offer your village? If a friend is going out of town, ask if they'd like you to water their plants or watch their pet.

- Be aware of time. Start wearing a watch and keeping a calendar. Listing all your responsibilities for the day is beneficial for even the most detail-oriented villager.

- Respond to texts and emails in a timely manner.

The Cheerleader Villager

The One Who Inspires

There are two ways of spreading light; to be /
The candle or the mirror that reflects it.
Edith Wharton

When we think of a cheerleader, we often think of someone whom we perceive to be artificially kind and peppy. Embracing a touch of that enthusiasm in our personal relationships can yield amazing results. I tell this to parents all the time: "Your kids need positive reinforcement!" And the same is true of your friends, your coworkers, and the members of your villages. Positive reinforcement doesn't mean being disingenuous. Instead, you are making a continual effort to encourage, uplift, and empower those close to you. And this doesn't mean you only cheer for someone when they're down—you also cheer in good times. In fact, sometimes, it's harder to put our egos aside to cheer someone on when they are accomplishing a goal. We might get caught up in questioning what we are accomplishing rather than concentrating on this member of our village.

Maybe you're like me, and enjoy cheering on everyone but yourself. As someone who is both a realist and an optimist, I do get excited when I reach a goal, but I also stay grounded. Recently a project that I was working on, which is still in the early stages, received great feedback. I told my best friend about it and said that I didn't want to get too excited—you know, don't count your chickens before they hatch? Instead of assuring me that I was being realistic and shouldn't get too excited, she said, "I'll be excited for you!" She believes I deserve happiness, even when I feel I don't. This was an example of my best friend being my cheerleader. Watching her excitement helped me see that we must celebrate each step in the process of accomplishing a goal.

So, how can you be a cheerleader? Yes, you can start by simply liking someone's social media post, but you should also aim to achieve larger goals as a cheerleader. This might sound like a broad statement, but it's important to stand by your villagers in times of success and times when they're being challenged. Like all villagers, a cheerleader takes on multiple forms. They are the ones who are cheering you on when you're at the twenty-fifth mile in a marathon, and they are also the people who come by to lift your spirits after a medical procedure. A cheerleader should be optimistic, realistic, and empathetic. The cheerleader is also able to see a situation from two different perspectives and note how both of you are feeling.

A cheerleader is curious, which shouldn't be confused with being nosy. They want to understand what a person needs, even if they don't fully understand every aspect of what the person is going through. For instance, if you're bolstering a friend who is in the middle of cancer treatment, they might not want to talk about every milestone they face, but you can still be there for them in small ways. You can simply show up and distract them when they are awaiting results. You might follow that person's lead and be there for them when they need you to be there, not when *you* want to be there. I mentioned that I received a wealth of well wishes when I was in the ER with kidney stones. A bunch of people sent a text saying, "Thinking of you." Each of those people was a cheerleader. They made me realize that although I was physically alone in the hospital, I wasn't alone at all.

When we talk about cheerleaders in this chapter, we are going to go beyond the thinking-of-you text. We'll go past the superficial "loud and animated" cheerleader stereotype and redefine what cheerleading means and how we can best help someone. Your words of encouragement can be quiet and not broadcast for the world to see. It doesn't have to be a grand gesture; it can be a small act that makes a huge difference in another person's life. In fact, there are many facets to a cheerleader, and they can serve various roles in your life. Unlike the other villagers, I feel we *all* have the potential to become cheerleader villagers.

In this chapter, we will work through a series of questions, quizzes, and tips to help us develop our inner cheerleader.

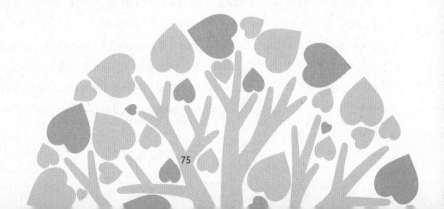

What Does the
Cheerleader Villager Look Like?

The cheerleader is the one who keeps you motivated. If you're going through a tough time, the cheerleader can be the friend who sits beside you on the couch watching reality TV even if they aren't a fan of it. (Okay, they don't have to be *that* selfless!) An effective cheerleader should think about what would make a villager happy and not what they themselves would enjoy. The cheerleader's actions should be thoughtful and well-intentioned. From sending flowers to dropping off a home-cooked meal, there are countless ways a cheerleader can make a challenging time easier.

Do you need a cheerleader if you're having a celebratory moment? Of course! What's the point of having a success in life if you can't share the excitement with your village? Let's say your friend is getting married—you can be their cheerleader by simply attending the event. I believe everyone who attends a wedding is essentially cheering on this new marriage (unless they get up during the vows and try to stop it!). Another way is to truly express happiness for the new couple. This doesn't mean you need to buy them a lavish gift. It means you somehow communicate that you're thinking about them that day. Consider (or ask) how you can make their day brighter.

Not everyone at a wedding is entirely happy for the bride and groom. Sometimes it's hard to be a cheerleader. There could be a guest at the wedding who is unmarried and wants to meet someone, or a guest who recently ended a relationship, and although they wish all the best for the couple, they might be too emotionally raw to *feel* happiness for the couple. Don't be disappointed with yourself if you can't be there for someone. This doesn't mean you won't be there for them forever. Recognize that at this moment, you aren't the best person to be a cheerleader for them.

If you're having a hard time deciphering what a cheerleader looks like, you might want to ask yourself these five questions to see if a person in your life can become a cheerleader in your village:

1   Do I feel comfortable sharing big decisions with this person even if I know they might not agree?

2   Do I feel nourished by our interactions, as opposed to drained?

3   Can I count on them to provide me with uncon-ditional support even if they can't support specific actions of mine?

4   Do I know that any advice they give me is entirely meant to support my best interest?

5   Can they uplift me when I'm low and help me sustain my highs?

Again, the questions in this book aren't easy ones to answer, and they might make you question certain relationships in your life. This is normal, and we should take the time to answer these questions thoughtfully. As I've mentioned, it would be helpful to dedicate a notebook to addressing all the questions and gut checks in the book. This notebook will serve as your bible for building your village.

Hopefully, after answering these questions, you will gain a better understanding of what a cheerleader looks like, but let's talk about their role in your village.

What Role Does the Cheerleader Villager Play?

You might be a private person and not comfortable sharing with others. Maybe you feel that a cheerleader villager isn't something you want or need. I say everyone needs a little encouragement now and then. We all have our own ways of processing issues, but, as we've learned, being solitary could be harmful to your health. You might also say that your dependable villager satisfies all your cheerleading needs, but be careful that you aren't overwhelming them. The cheerleader doesn't have to be close to you but will support you in ways that make you feel stronger and happier.

Maybe you believe you are your own cheerleader. If so, that's fantastic. Yet I still think having a cheer squad is something that can enhance your life. Even if you think you don't need or want a cheerleader in your life, please do this quick exercise.

EXERCISE

Do I Need a Cheer Squad?

1. *Are you pursuing a goal, either big or small? If the latter, does it have multiple benchmarks occuring over time?*

2. *Are you going through any milestones in your life?*

3. *Are you a caregiver for another person?*

4. *Are you considering making any changes in your life?*

5. *Are you silently struggling with a problem?*

If you answered yes to any of those questions, which I'm sure you did, then you would benefit from having someone on your cheer squad. Let's focus on question number four. This question stands out because it's vague. This is intentional. Life is all about change, and to get the most out of life, we need to think about the future and how we envision ourselves in it. When we take time to reflect on our next stages in life, we inevitably learn that changes are in order. The reason I'm focusing on this question is that *I truly believe we all need a cheerleader in our lives.* The cheer squad is especially helpful when we're undergoing major changes, but they are also there to support us through the small ones.

We should also acknowledge that life might also throw us unexpected changes. Some of them are positive. We cannot know how big the change will be when we first meet a new friend, or find love, or are referred for a great job. Other changes aren't necessarily positive at first but are catalysts for advancement. I know two people who lost their jobs and then decided to pivot their careers. I watched as people cheered them on during their career change and continued to do so when these two found success in their new careers during their forties. It's fulfilling to rally around someone through a challenging time and see them succeed. Other times, we cheer for someone and it doesn't work out. This is okay. The fact that you stand by a person through the challenging time and still consistently show that you're a supportive presence is enough to make a difference in that person's life.

Earlier I mentioned that by simply attending a wedding, you play the role of a cheerleader. This same thought applies to people who attend a funeral. Yes, a funeral is a somber event, and you should be respectful and reserved. No, a funeral is not a place to be overtly upbeat. And yes, it might appear strange that I define guests at both a wedding and a funeral as cheerleaders, but I do. When my Nana died, I was utterly destroyed. There are no words to express that intense grief. My best friends remarked that they had never seen me that sad. They were concerned. They were witnessing a low they'd not encountered before. Truthfully, I wasn't familiar with that side of myself, either. I hadn't lost anyone I loved as deeply as my Nana. She was my biggest cheerleader, and I was hers. This was a selfless, loving woman who dedicated her life to family and whose legacy of kindness inspires me each day.

During this time, I had to relearn how to be happy again. The friends who stood by me by showing up and helping me find my way back to my cheerful self, let me grieve but also served as reflections of who I had been and was going to be again. This seemed impossible in the days and weeks following my Nana's passing, when all the life seemed to drain from me. As you may have guessed, I'm a high-energy person, but in the aftermath of grief I was lethargic and unsocial. I put my career on the back burner, and I wasn't as focused in general. My cheerleaders during that time helped me by sending me messages, making plans with me when I didn't even want to get out of bed, and reminding me to laugh and enjoy my life. They helped me pay tribute to my grandmother and taught me to remember her but also to keep going.

There are numerous ways a cheerleader can be part of your village. A number of the qualities this person displays are seen in the other villagers. You've probably noticed that some of the dependable villager actions—like delivering a meal when someone is ill—are also cheerleader actions. One aspect that differentiates the cheerleader from the other roles is the subtle optimistic quality of all their interactions. This isn't to say they are delusional or employing magical thinking, but they can somehow identify the silver linings when you can't even see what's in front of you. The cheerleader is truly thinking of you and not themself—something everyone needs in their lives.

After I paused the IVF, I was blindsided by my body's hormonal reaction. We hear people talk about "baby blues" and postpartum depression, but few people talk about the emotional effects after IVF treatment. I didn't feel like myself, and there seemed nothing I could do to change that. My family and friends were again concerned by my new behavior. What really scared me was not knowing how long it would last. I yearned to feel like my old self. I mourned the upbeat person I once was. During this time, a friend sent me a text letting me know that she couldn't fix what was going on with me, but she would text me every day. Each text said the equivalent of "you will get through this" or "this will pass." She was right. Her constant messages showed me that a cheerleader can see in you what you can't. The cheerleader villager does not have an easy job. It's hard to see a friend suffering and know there is little you can do to solve their problems. And yet, it's an endlessly rewarding role to help others get through their troubles.

How Can I Be a Cheerleader Villager?

Admittedly, the term *cheerleader* is something of a misnomer, since the focus should not be on acting *cheerfully* but rather on acting *supportively*. You can be a cheerleader villager even if you disagree with a friend's decision. You should not feel as though you can't express your opinion. But you can do so in a way that aims not to hurt but to help. Make it clear that you still support the person even if you don't support the decision itself. Let them know you will continue to provide that support in spite of any choices they make. Remember, at the end of the day, the members of your village are leading lives different than your own, and part of being a cheerleader is learning when to cheer.

Some people instinctively know how to lift someone's spirits; it's second nature. Those people will tell you that it's easier to do so for others than for yourself. Or at least, that's how I feel. I love cheering on my fellow villagers. It makes me feel great to help others, and I find that being a cheerleader is the most accessible of all the village roles. We don't have to commit a large amount of time, and we can vary our level of intensity for cheering. We can send a text, or we can physically show up for someone. Other village roles may require more time and commitment. This means you can definitely be a cheerleader in multiple circles, as long as you budget your time wisely.

Easy Ways to Cheer

Don't know how to cheer? You can start with small acts of caring support and graduate to larger ones. Being a cheerleader doesn't have to be a full-time job! There are easy ways that you can nurture your inner cheerleader and support the members of your villages!

Here are a few tips.

Send Messages of Encouragement

A simple message might seem small, but oftentimes it's the little acts of compassion and love that really keep us going. Be sure to check in with members of your community often, and make it clear that you are there for them, particularly if they're going through a rough time. Remember that a small message can have a big impact. Be specific! In theatrical tradition you wouldn't tell an actor "good luck," you'd say "break a leg!" Be sensitive to their situation and needs. Go the extra mile when sharing words of encouragement, because attention to such details shows that you care.

Care Packages

In sororities we have a tradition called "Bigs/Littles" where an older "sister" takes a younger one under her wing and provides her with a series of welcoming gifts. I love this tradition, because it's about welcoming somebody into a community and helping them create a home. When I moved into the house I live in now, I felt that same love and community when my neighbors greeted me with small presents and baked goods! Making a care package for a villager can be a wonderful way to be cheerleader. For instance, if a friend recently had a baby, consider putting together a package of their favorite snacks instead of typical baby gifts, since I know from experience that shopping with a baby can be HARD WORK (and it's difficult to get in a full meal between the baby's feedings!). You don't even need a reason to provide somebody with a care package or a small token of how much you appreciate them. Bringing somebody flowers or a coffee can show them that you're thinking about them and that you care. Honestly, I should retitle this chapter "The Careleader Villager," since cheerleading is truly the art of caring.

Be Honest

Honesty is the best policy! Brutal honesty might seem antithetical to cheerleading, but like our parents told us as children, nothing good comes of lying. While a little white lie might not hurt every now and then, it's important to share our honest opinions with the people we care about. If a friend comes to you questioning their career path and contemplating quitting their job, you do not have to support this move in order to serve as a cheerleader. The best cheerleaders know when to take a step back and *support* the members of their villages without *enabling* them. Remember that cheerleaders are watching the game, too, in order to know when it's the right time to cheer. If you feel a friend is making a decision that is not in their best interest, it's your job as a cheerleader to speak up. Do so with love, compassion, and grace, but also make your voice heard. You hope that you won't be cheering for your friend as they lose but as they win, and sometimes it's good to pause and strategize in order to achieve that goal.

These are a few ideas to get you started. Now, go out and cheer for someone!

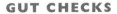

GUT CHECKS

- Do you feel it's easier to cheer for someone who is struggling rather than to cheer for someone who has a success?

- When was the last time you were truly happy for someone?

- Do you have the emotional energy to cheer someone on?

ACTION STEPS

- Think of a friend who may be feeling overwhelmed. Create a care package for them. It can even be a digital care package, like an electronic gift card to a local coffee shop if they are burning the candle at both ends. Be creative!

- Find a friend who could use a smile. Send them a handwritten note or a postcard describing all the qualities you admire in them. When I was undergoing fertility treatment, a friend sent me a card noting all the things she loved about me, and it both warmed my heart and helped me through that challenging time.

- Be generous to a stranger. Find a local charity where you can donate gifts, food, or clothes, and cheer on people who are in need.

The Communicator Villager

The One Who Communicates Effectively

You must do the thing you think you cannot do.

Eleanor Roosevelt

For years, parents have reached out to me to help them build villages. Within their requests, I noticed a pattern—they all had folks in their lives who could help them, but these parents didn't know how to ask for what they needed. But why is asking so difficult? I had a discussion on social media with Nina Spears, the founder of Baby Chick, on this subject. Nina helps expectant and new moms plan for prenatal and postnatal care, and we talked about the challenges new parents face when it comes to putting together a village. We agreed that even when we can communicate our needs to ourselves, we often find it impossible to tell others that we are in need. Why is this so difficult? Are we afraid people will think we are weak? Or do we want to project a flawless image of ourselves? Asking for assistance is essential when building real relationships. If we can't call upon our friends to help us out, then they aren't our friends.[1]

I believe that people want to ask for help, but they may lack the language to communicate their needs. To attach words to a feeling seems basic, but it isn't easy. People spend years in therapy trying to figure out their own needs. I'll add that it's okay for you to not always know what you need at any given moment. This is where the communicator can help. In this chapter we'll address how you can become a better communicator and how you can find an effective communicator villager.

If you go by stereotypes of what we believe a communicator should look like, you might find yourself challenged during your search. For instance, we might think that someone who talks a lot is a great communicator, but that's not necessarily the case. Yes, talking is a form of communicating, but talking doesn't always result in successfully communicating needs. Sometimes, we don't even know what we want to communicate. In fact, one of the best ways to find a communicator is not to search for a talker but to look for a listener. A listener is one of the most effective communicators. They are also often skilled at reading people's nonverbal cues.

The first step to finding an effective communicator is knowing yourself and what you want. To some, this might seem indulgent and mildly narcissistic, but it's exactly the opposite. Once you've done the work and figured out what you want, you will be able to help others. This is not to say that we all have to play the role of a communicator villager, but it is a skill that we must nurture in ourselves before we do so in others.

The tricky part is that we all communicate differently. Some of us, like me, are outside processors. This means I like to talk out my problems and even (Beware! You might judge me!) talk to myself when I'm attempting to solve an issue in my life. I find that talking out my problems helps me understand my thoughts. Of course, this is why I often talk to myself first, because if I'm having an issue with someone else, I don't want to hurt their feelings. I want to figure out the best way to approach the situation. I like to rehearse what I'll say, so that I am communicating thoughtfully.

So, let's start communicating! We'll find out what makes a great communicator and how we can brush up on our communication skills. We will use quizzes, exercises, and other steps to help you identify your needs and discover the communicator villager in yourself and the people you choose to be in your village.

What Does the Communicator Villager Look Like?

As we discussed before, a communicator isn't the loudest person in the room but the most thoughtful. This means you're looking for someone who can understand the needs of others. The communicator can take diverse forms. For instance, it can be someone who gets their point across through writing. When a friend of mine was undergoing treatment for cancer, one of her villagers sent out a weekly email letting people know about her progress and how we could help her. This person effectively expressed my friend's needs so she could focus on recovering. Or the communicator could be someone who reads your nonverbal cues and can help you when you don't even know what you need. Do you have a friend who brings you flowers when they see you're having a hard day? That would be a communicator who can read nonverbal cues. You can't expect the communicator to be a mind reader, though. I actively try to avoid miscommunication. I express myself and don't let anything build up.

As you can see, the role has a wide range, and you might even find that you could use two communicators in your village, but I'll talk more about that later. Let's start your search for this vital villager by asking what type of communicator you need. Since this isn't always a straightforward task, here are a few questions that will help guide you as you search for a communicator.

What Type of Communicator Do I Need?

1 **What type of village are you creating?** Do you think you'll need help getting the message of the community across to others? For instance, if this is a secondary village needed to produce an event like a fundraiser, do you need someone who can send texts or emails to the group? If this is a primary village, do you need someone who can help you communicate your basic needs? For instance, I have a friend who can tell when I'm hangry and doesn't listen to a word I say until I've had a bite to eat. That's a more subtle communicator, but it still fulfills that role in the village.

2   What do you think makes someone an effective communicator? Why?

3   What role do you see this villager having in your community? Do you think you might need more than one communicator?

These are a few questions you should answer before you embark on your search. As I always say, the more you know about what you want, the more likely you are to find it. Also, this is a role that might not be as easily defined as the dependable villager or the cheerleader. It's also a role that might overlap or work in tandem with the organizer villager, which we will discuss in the next chapter. However, even if you think *you* are the best communicator in the world, you still need a communicator.

When I was running my own company, I understood the importance of a good communications team. Even though I love to write, I knew I couldn't produce all the press releases and other materials needed to get my company's mission across to customers and potential clients. You want to give others a chance to fulfill their roles, and you shouldn't take on too many roles yourself. This is true in the business world and in your personal life. We need to understand our limitations and respect the talents of others. Also, it's important to showcase other people's voices.

When choosing a communicator, find someone who won't try to push their agenda. Make sure they are there to serve as a mirror for the group. They should express the needs of others, not just their own needs. This is an important role within your community, and you ought to cast this role wisely. How do you know you chose the right person? Here's a quiz.

Communicator Quiz

Answer yes or no to the following questions:

1   **Is this person capable of seeing other perspectives?**

2   **Do they ask thoughtful questions?**

3   **Will they have your best interests in mind?**

4   **Can they succinctly explain a problem?**

5   **Have they proven to be a good listener?**

If you answered yes to all five of these questions, you have found a potential candidate for this role. Don't confuse the role of a communicator with that of a spokesperson. This villager isn't someone who is chosen to speak for the group at all times, but someone who can reach out to others when the village is in need of extra hands or when all are collectively working together to get a task done. They could also help the villagers communicate with one another. This means you should choose someone who is usually even-tempered, is reasonable, and tends to get along with others. Historically, we have also seen skilled communicators use their abilities to stir up trouble or incite bad behavior. We don't want to select someone who might cause tension within the group. But, this doesn't mean the communicator villager should be a pushover. They aren't someone who is easily swayed but rather a strong, well-intentioned person who understands how to tactfully address a plethora of situations.

I've never been afraid of leadership. Throughout my youth, I took on leadership positions at school and was president of the student council, editor of the high school newspaper, and so on. As I grew older, I ran my own company. After sitting on panels with executives, I noticed a common denominator around people who knew how to communicate successfully. If you strip it back, it's all about curiosity. However, being curious is only one step in the process of cementing relationships and learning how to communicate with others. Although I was curious about others, it took time to get to know people and establish business relationships. I had to be present in conversation and establish trust with new people in my life.

What Role Does the Communicator Villager Play?

We've addressed what the communicator looks like, but now we'll see how they participate in village life. Since there are numerous ways people communicate, I suggest that people look for two different communicator villagers—one who will help them emotionally and another who will serve a more practical role. You can think of this as a bonus villager you are welcoming into your community. I mentioned an example of the practical communicator earlier in the chapter: the person who sent out emails when my friend was undergoing cancer treatment. On the other hand, my friend who always knows when I'm hungry and forces me to eat is an "emotional" communicator.

Each person's emotional language feels and sounds different. Put in the time and effort to discover the ways other people express their emotions. It's like a game of poker: you don't just pay attention to the cards you're dealt; you spend an equal amount of time watching the players' expressions and seeing how they process the cards they're holding in their hands. Of course, in poker, the best players try not to reveal any clues about the hand they're playing. In real life, though, it's harmful to display that behavior. This is when we need an emotional communicator who can reveal what we are hiding from ourselves and others.

Let's say you've gotten upset over something relatively benign. Instead of reacting to your distress, this emotional communicator might open a discussion on why you are engaging in toxic behavior. An emotional communicator is ideal for diffusing tense situations within a village. Of course, you shouldn't treat this person like the community therapist, because that wouldn't be fair to them. Another thing to be mindful of is that since this person can communicate, they also hold a lot of power in your group. You can't let them speak for you; rather, they should speak *with* you. Make sure they have your best intentions in mind and that they aren't crossing any boundaries.

Types of Communicators

If you're looking for more concrete examples of how a communicator villager fits in your community, here are a few types of communicator villagers:

The Writer

A writer can establish written communication for the group. If they're part of a secondary village like a school club or workplace, maybe they create the newsletter. Or they're someone who sends a text when you're feeling down. They use writing to express their emotions and wants.

The Speaker

Who doesn't love a good talker? However, we don't need someone who only tell us jokes or makes insincere statements. A speaker can facilitate productive conversations between all the people in the group. They also might be skilled at making a toast or giving a speech.

The Listener

The listener isn't someone who is shy or isn't necessarily a big talker. In fact, I find plenty of talkers to be great listeners. The listener not only absorbs what you're saying and reads your nonverbal cues but also processes this information and uses it to help you and others. They can often tell if someone is in a bad mood, and they know when to speak and when to be quiet.

The Peacemaker

The peacemaker knows that conflict shouldn't be avoided, but it also shouldn't be allowed to sour anyone's relationships. The peacemaker helps alleviate issues within the group and lets people voice their opinions. Earlier in the book I discussed how people have different, often conflicting values. The peacemaker respects everyone's values, even if they don't share them. Similar to the accepting villager, they can meet people where they are and not where they want them to be.

The Leader

I debated using the word *leader*. I don't like to define anyone as a leader when it comes to a village. Even if you're the one creating the support circle, it doesn't make you the leader of it. However, I use the term leader here to define someone who can get everyone's attention and let the community's voice be heard.

Did I leave any communicators out? If you think so, please contact me. I hope you know that I want to help you out with your village. In fact, while writing this book I was inspired to start a virtual village group on social media. That might seem like a small step, and I haven't had it for long, but I am absolutely loving this group. Each day, I awake to find new members, and I am inspired by the comments they post in the group. Since this is a digital group, it's based on written communication. This means we are all playing the role of communicator in the virtual village. I take on the main role in this virtual space because I'm the one generating the content and questions. I point this out because everyone in the village has a voice that needs to be heard. Even if someone isn't broadcasting messages to the entire group, their words still hold equal weight.

This virtual group is a great way to find someone who might be a communicator for your village. It's also a space where folks can ask me questions and respond to the book. I'd be more than happy to open any discussion about the book on social media, so reach out to me! You don't have to be part of the virtual village if you don't want to, but feel free to send me a message.

Okay, let's stop talking about the virtual village and get back to creating yours. Aren't you on the hunt for a communicator? I'd like you to take a minute to write down all the qualities you believe a communicator should have. I wish I could see your list! Now I want to share what I think are signs of a consciously compassionate communicator. Later in the book, I devote an entire chapter to the art of being mindfully compassionate. Being compassionate is an essential quality for every villager, but it's fundamental for the communicator.

Signs of a Consciously Compassionate Communicator

- Consciously compassionate communicators ask questions rather than making statements.

- They don't criticize.

- They open a dialogue with others in a comfortable environment.

- They are curious.

- They don't try to convince others that their views are the right ones.

- They can see multiple perspectives on a situation.

- They are understanding.

These are a few qualities that I came up with after years of being part of various villages. I like to keep notes on the groups I'm part of and to see the types of people who have been cast for roles in those groups. I think back to the years that I was employed as a nanny. Since children's voices are often ignored, I was consistently the communicator villager in those networks. There were times I had to advocate for a child and let their voice be heard. As you might expect, this wasn't always easy—I think we all know how hard it can be to talk about a child with their parent. However, I didn't offer my opinion when I communicated their child's needs, I just let the family know my understanding of what the child was feeling. Please don't let your beliefs alter someone else's words. The communicator is a messenger, not a dictator or a boss. They are a friend who helps the group flourish through talking and other forms of communication.

How Can I Be a Communicator Villager?

I know this is going to sound counterproductive, but the first step to becoming a communicator villager is to stop talking. Spend a day observing everyone around you. Take a deep look at your relationships and your habits of communication. Do the following exercise to see how you communicate with the people in your life.

EXERCISE

What Type of Communicator Am I?

- *Do you journal?*

- *Do you feel you need to unpack issues through dialogue?*

- *Think about the last interaction you had with someone. It could even have been a casual interaction. Did you feel heard? Why?*

- *When have you felt your words weren't heard? Why?*

- *Do you get annoyed if someone talks over you?*

- *Do you find yourself wanting to speak when someone else speaks?*

There are no right or wrong answers to these questions, but they're good prompts for opening a discussion with yourself on how you communicate. Even if you think you're the strongest communicator, it's vital to examine the ways you speak to people. Of course, we don't communicate the same way with everyone in our lives. For example, you aren't going to talk to your child the same way you talk to your boss. This sounds obvious, but sometimes we forget the importance of thoughtful communication.

We should also be mindful of any bad habits we have when we communicate and take steps to address them. If you know that you're hot tempered, find ways to calm down before engaging in a conversation. Another issue some people have is speaking when someone else is talking. I come from a large Italian family, where our dinners are lively and filled with several conversations at once. I love this, but I know that's not everyone's scene. You don't want to overwhelm the people you are communicating with. Since I'm guilty of such bad habits at times, I came up with a list of tips for being a thoughtful communicator.

As someone who spent years as a nanny, teaching multiple children how to interact in various social situations, I think about the rules I taught them. There were constant reminders to say please and thank you, of course, but that's rather basic. It became more complicated when the child had a conflict with another, or they wanted something they couldn't have. These were times when I'd have to show the kids the proper way to interact with others. Here are some tips that I've learned over the years in both my personal and professional life. I refer to them frequently, and I hope you find them helpful too.

Tips for Being a Thoughtful Communicator

- Try to be mindful about the time you choose to have a conversation with someone. For example, don't schedule a discussion for late in the day, when members of the village could be tired. Make sure it's a good communication time for everyone involved.

- Never speak for someone else unless they've requested you to.

- Be prepared; try to write a few points you'd like to make before you address the village.

- Don't enter an argument expecting to win. Always try to forgive the other person if they apologize.

- Be open-minded. Even if you have issues with the one(s) you are addressing, listen to them and try to be reasonable.

Those are a few thoughts I keep in mind when I'm trying to communicate. As I said, I'm someone who likes to talk things out, but I know a bunch of people who like to journal. Of course you can do both! Becoming a good communicator, whatever its form, takes time and effort. Learn how to listen, and think about how others might perceive a situation. All too often, we limit ourselves and only think about how we see things. As I said before, when I start to feel limited in my thinking, I revisit the idea that we all have a specific set of values. Perhaps I am struggling to communicate with someone because our values aren't aligned. In this situation, we both must understand that it's okay for others to prioritize different values. A good way to figure out if you're unable to communicate due to differing value sets is to ask questions of both yourself and the one(s) with whom you're communicating.

Once you distance yourself from the emotional aspect of communication and try to figure out why you're not communicating successfully, you'll begin to strengthen your skills. Then you'll be able to have deeper and more meaningful relationships.

Another reason people struggle with communication is due to their fear of rejection. Being rejected doesn't feel good, but it's essential for growth. Some people fear rejection so intensely that they find themselves doing anything to avoid it. Here's an example: I know people who are afraid to start a conversation with someone—even at an event as benign and low-stakes as a casual dinner party—because they don't want to be rejected, or they're afraid they'll stand out for the wrong reason.

During a conversation with a newly single friend, she revealed to me that she didn't know how to be on her own. Since I've spent so many years as the single gal and seemed used to doing things by myself, she had reached out to me for advice. I told her that I had not considered how being on your own might feel awkward or scary. Although it's not the most natural thing for everyone to do, I am comfortable attending events on my own. I chalk this up to the fact that I love public speaking. I know it's the number-one fear for countless folks, but I was born to stand in front of a microphone, and I rarely shy away from attention. This isn't to say that I don't have other fears—I do. (My number-one fear is elevators.) I helped my friend navigate her life as a single. I suggested she ask people questions and pay attention to how much people enjoy talking about themselves. If you express curiosity about others, you are more likely to communicate successfully.

GUT CHECKS

- Do you remember the last conversation you had? Try to pinpoint at least two things that person told you during that interaction.

- Have you ever understood what someone was feeling without them telling you in words? How? And how did you react?

- How does your position in life reflect the way you talk to people? If you're a people manager, do you find your style of communication more direct than most?

ACTION STEPS

- Start keeping a "communication log." Note who you talk to, how you communicate with them (text, email, in person, phone), and how each interaction makes you feel.

- Each day for one week, contact a different person you haven't spoken to in a while. Check in and ask them how they are doing. Reaching out is the first step to communicating.

- Ask people how they like to communicate. Do they prefer texts, emails, or the phone? When you learn people's preferences, you have a better chance of active engagement.

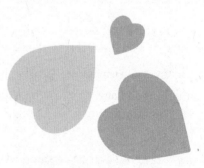

The Organizer Villager

The One Who Organizes

For every minute spent organizing, an hour is earned.

Anonymous

I have a neighbor who knows how to plan anything, and I'm not exaggerating. She has lived in my town her entire life, and she spent that time cultivating resources. To me, it feels like she is the town's guardian angel. I recall when another neighbor's house burnt down, this woman immediately organized emergency assistance. She gathered donations ranging from clothes to toothbrushes and other essentials. She enlisted people in the town to help the family resettle. See what I mean? Guardian angel. And she doesn't even want credit for her good deeds. Everything she does for others is done quietly, without expecting a thank you, a reward, or special acknowledgment. Her generosity is inspiring, but what is even more impressive is the way she skillfully organizes these acts of kindness.

And then there's the family friend who might rival my neighbor in her stealthy organizational skills. When my grandfather, whom we affectionately called Papa, died, this friend immediately asked how she could help. Before I could even open my mouth to respond, she wanted to know if we had anyone flying in from out of town, because she'd pick them up at the airport. Like my neighbor, this friend humbly and generously helps. She displays several qualities of the villagers described in this book (her offers of help are dependable, and she's a good communicator), but her main strength is as an organizer. I see her as the conductor of an orchestra, and every note is perfectly executed.

I started this chapter with the above two examples because I want you to see the power of the organizer villager. This person can get things done. All organizer villagers recognize strengths in others and know how to cultivate those skills so they can run a successful support system. There are different types of organizer villagers, from those who serve as hands-on planners to others whose skills are more conceptual in nature. In fact, in picking up this book and wanting to start a village, you are playing the role of a conceptual organizer villager. You're striving to create a productive community and you're conceptualizing that world before you cast the roles.

I should note that there are also times when you may need to hire an organizer villager. For instance, my sister is getting married, and she hired a wedding planner. Of late I've noticed a trend of people hiring planners for a variety of life events. From life coaches to home organizers, there is a need to help people out in order aspects of their lives. Remember in the last chapter when I talked about my discussion with Nina Spears? She helps expectant parents plan for their baby's arrival.

Yes, you can hire someone if you are part of a secondary village and need help putting together a party or another event. However, the organizer villager has a more varied role in your primary village. They bring energy into the community and are skilled in building relationships and drawing together different groups of people. One of my friends has a knack for reading personalities and connecting compatible people. When I moved back to the suburbs, she introduced me to people she thought I'd get along with.

In the business world, connecting with people is essential for establishing yourself in your industry. Networking events can put you in touch with potential colleagues and friends. I met one friend through the National Organization of Women Business Owners. If you tell her what type of person you need for your business, she will find a bunch of names for you. I credit this to her warm and inviting personality. She asks questions and makes whomever she's talking to feel like the most important person in the room. Her first instinct is to help others. I think of her when I hear the saying attributed to Édith Piaf, "When you reach the top, you should remember to send the elevator back down for the others." She always sends the elevator down.

What type of organizer do you need, and how can you find them? And what do they look like in your village? We will discuss how to search for an organizer and the best way to cultivate organizational skills in yourself. Through questions, quizzes, and action steps we will cast a villager for this role and start getting things done!

What Does the Organizer Villager Look Like?

The organizer has important roles in the village. Yes, they help the group get things done, but this isn't their sole purpose. Think about the diverse ways we organize. For instance, some of us like to organize social events. As I mentioned, I know a few people who are skilled at connecting others. This type of organizer is essential if you're moving to a new place and trying to build a village from scratch. This person doesn't have to be a potential friend, and they need not even be part of the community you create, but they can connect you with people you want to add to your village. What are this person's characteristics? You might recognize them as someone who loves to plan events. Do you have a coworker who organizes a "Thirsty Thursday" happy hour? Or a friend who runs a book club?

You don't even have to leave the house to find this type of villager. We are growing ever more accustomed to socializing online—these sorts of groups have stuck around long after the stay-at-home mandates from COVID-19 were lifted. Ideally your initial organizer villager finds joy in bringing people together. However, if you feel that you can't find this type of person, you might want to join a few existing organizations that offer events. These are great places to meet new people.

If you're already part of a community, like a local charity, you'll see another type of organizer in action—the one who knows how to accomplish things. This is the person you probably think of when you imagine an organizer. This type of individual leads committees and can delegate responsibilities without dictating orders—one who orchestrates the event. Such people are vital for any group because they keep track of all that needs to be carried out. If you're part of a secondary parenting village, you can easily spot the organizers: they are the ones who put together carpools, group play dates, and so on. In secondary villages like these, identifying the organizers is a bit easier than in a primary village. The role of the organizer is a bit more subtle in a primary village. Perhaps they are someone who keeps track of birthdays and plans holiday get-togethers.

Vetting a Potential Organizer

How do you know someone would make a good organizer? Here are some questions to ask to spot a potential organizer villager. Take out your notebook and list a few people you might consider casting for this role. Then answer these three questions about each person:

1 **Are they flexible?**

2 **Can they communicate well?**

3 **Can they find and nurture skills in others?**

The reason I ask if they're flexible is that many people think organized people are necessarily rigid, and this just isn't true. We shouldn't limit ourselves to thinking that because someone likes order, they are unable to process chaos. I find the best organizers to be versatile and able to roll with changes. These are people who like to keep things moving along and know how to motivate others to get work done. This means we ought to find someone who knows how to communicate. This isn't to say that the organizer villager should also be the communicator villager, though as I mentioned, several of these roles overlap. I've said that the organizer is the "conductor" of the village. In an orchestra, the conductor doesn't need to know how to play all the instruments, but they need to know how to listen and how to read music. The organizer, in turn, needs to know how to read people. They also need to know how to nurture the skills they recognize in others, so the village can create beautiful music.

What Role Does the Organizer Villager Play?

There are numerous ways one can be organized, from the person who has a tidy house to the one who drafts detailed to-do lists for emergency response in the community. When it comes to finding someone to fill the organizer role, you might want to search for a person who satisfies a few of the traits of organizers (page 109–11), or potentially all of them! Again, you're the one in control. You are the creator and should have an idea of what you want the village to look like. If you're building your primary village, you're looking for someone who can help get the village together for events. If you're creating a secondary village, you might want an organizer who will keep a spreadsheet of responsibilities for the village or create a sign-up sheet for an event.

When I was a nanny, I noted that the moms were often the organizer villagers. They would alert me to all the obligations each child had, from tennis lessons to dance practice, and would send me the schedules. In my business world, I found that office managers and people in other production-related jobs were strong organizers. In my personal life and primary village, our organizer makes sure we have birthday celebrations, cocktail nights, and other events on our calendar. As I thought about the villages in my life, I came up with types of organizers that we might want in our communities.

Types of Organizers

Here are six organizer roles you could potentially cast for your village:

Social Organizer

Do you love to arrange social events? A social organizer might run networking groups or be an online moderator. This type of organizer could have a superficial role in your primary or even secondary village, but they're experts at getting the right mix of people together. It's important to have a few organizers like this in your life because they help you to meet other people, which you need to do when growing your village. If you can't find such a person, you can substitute this social organizer with an established religious or community group.

Technical Organizer

No, a technical organizer doesn't have to know how to do tech-related things like answer questions about your smartphone, but they understand what needs to be done, step by step, to accomplish a goal. In certain cases, you might hire this type of organizer (like my sister's wedding planner). They are skilled at creating spreadsheets, drafting contact lists, and making sure the technical details aren't overlooked. An example of a technical organizer would be the person who sets up a meal train when a villager is sick and unable to cook their own food.

Emergency Organizer

Even if someone is super organized and can put together an event or send out a newsletter to keep everyone in the village informed, they might not be at their best when an emergency arises. Not everyone is suited to be at your side when something bad has happened, and that's okay. On the other hand, I know some people who only reveal their organization skills when an emergency arises. This type of organizer might normally play another role in your primary and secondary villages and only hold this role when it's needed.

Conceptual Organizer

Everyone who is reading this book is a conceptual organizer. You have the concept for your village and are laying the groundwork to create it through the quizzes, questions, action steps, and gut checks. If you have an idea of how you'd like your primary and secondary communities to function and how you'd like to be part of others' villages, that makes you a conceptual organizer! However, you will also want someone else who is good at coming up with ideas when organizing an event or creating a new project. This type of villager offers suggestions, but they might not be skilled at executing them. They're the dreamers, the creatives. They need to be paired with a producer, which is usually the technical organizer.

The Original Organizer

Do you have a friend who loves to organize their closet, pantry, or glove compartment? Someone who is never late and can seamlessly arrange events? They might have the skills of the technical organizer and be as socially savvy as a cruise director. They can pretty much organize everything from origin to conclusion. Let's just say that organizing is their superpower. If you're fortunate enough to come across this multitalented organizer, they might wear many organizer hats within your support system.

Support Team

The organizer is one villager who can't work alone. The other members of the village form the support team, usually led by the organizer. Since the organizer is skilled at seeing the strengths in others, they can assign roles within the support team. A good organizer knows how to motivate a group and make them feel seen, heard, and appreciated.

These are a few organizers I wanted to highlight. You may have an idea of a specific type of organizer that you need for your village. This is great. However, I advise you to be flexible when searching for an organizer. Just because your friend has a messy car or house doesn't mean they can't get the job done.

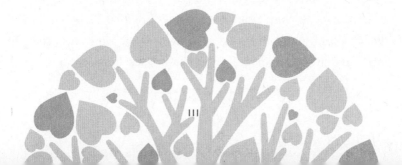

How Can I Be an Organizer Villager?

I would like to think I'm organized. I make lists. I like routine. I'm an obsessive planner and researcher when it comes to every aspect of my life. That said, I am able to leave room for error and creativity. I learned the importance of making space for possible errors when I started in the business world. As I mentioned earlier, there was a period when I had to seek out a consultant to help my business when it was struggling. I was devastated, but I also learned a lot about myself and my business. As I conferred with the consultant—who was able to take everything I had organized, evaluate it, and point out where the business could improve—I realized that even a diligently organized person can make mistakes.

So, when people think that I am rigid because I'm organized, I explain that it is possible to be both organized and flexible. Business taught me that I had to be nimble. Yes, I had my day planned, and then things came up and I went with whatever the day brought me. I allowed the events of the day to unfold. Of course, I completed priority tasks first and picked up the pieces later. That said, this wasn't something that was instinctual. When I first started my business, at times I was indeed rigid and had tunnel vision, but I learned that being flexible is the most important part of being organized.

The organizer is commonly the founder of the village, but you don't have to keep this role as your circle grows. You are going to be casting several roles, and you can abandon the role of organizer when you start filling your village. This reminds me of when I started my company. Since it was something that I had built, I was used to controlling every aspect of the way the work was produced and the staff was managed. In addition, I felt I needed to be tough because I'm a woman, and I wanted to be heard. This resulted in me micromanaging every aspect of the company. I felt an enormous pressure because I knew if my company failed, my employees wouldn't be able to support their families. However, being a micromanager backfired on me. Big surprise, right? Actually, I was doing everyone a disservice. I wasn't allowing the staff to spread their wings and nourish their talents. The consultant I hired did a holistic evaluation of my company, and as a result I learned how to run my company more efficiently. The consultant told me that you can't work *on* the business and *in* the business at the same time. I let an invaluable employee take over responsibilities that I shouldn't have been managing, and it allowed the company to grow. Basically, I had to reorganize myself as well as my business.

Organization isn't all about business, though. I often think about the role I've played as organizer in many people's villages. At this point in my life, I've been in fifteen wedding parties. I'm honored to be part of these happy occasions, and I have tried to make each one memorable. When friends ask me to be in their wedding parties, they know I'm hyper-organized and that if I'm charged with doing the work, I get it done. I also like to do it with flair. These event experiences have taught me the importance of being organized—it can help keep the focus on their important day—with love and joy instead of anxiety about logistics.

So, what happens if you're not organized? For instance, I have a friend who lacks organizational skills when it comes to physical items. She stresses when packing for a trip and can spend an afternoon searching for a single item in her closet. Yet she is a great social organizer, and she is extremely successful in other aspects of her life, many of which involve being detail oriented. The truth is we are all organized in different ways, but we have different organizational behaviors. That messy friend has an amazing memory and doesn't miss deadlines or appointments. So, if she wanted to join a village, she might be the organizer who remembers special events or birthdays and anniversaries.

As you can see there are numerous ways in which you can be an organizer. Here is an exercise that I developed to help you reflect on what type of organizer you might be.

What Type of Organizer Am I?

Answer these questions to figure out your organizational strengths:

- *How are your time management skills?*

- *Describe the last time you organized something. It can be small. Go into detail about that process. Did you plan before you started this project? Do you remember your first step?*

- *Do you keep to-do lists?*

- *What does delegation mean to you?*

- *Can you think of a time you felt overwhelmed? Were you reluctant to ask for help?*

Five Tips for Becoming a Better Organizer

1 Be able to let go and have someone else take control.

2 Think of ways you can adjust your routine.

3 Declutter both your home and your mind.

4 Take small steps to avoid procrastination.

5 Find inspiration from others.

These are tips that have helped throughout my personal and professional life. Once you incorporate some or all of them into your life, you will be able to become more organized. It isn't something that will happen overnight, but you will see concrete changes. I think the major change you might want to make is to let go and let someone else take the lead. I know when I try to organize every aspect of my life it usually backfires on me. This is why having another organizer in your village is so important.

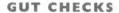

GUT CHECKS

- Do you feel you take on too many projects? Describe an example.

- What is a current goal you have? Name one step you need to take toward achieving that goal.

- Do you rely on others to get things done?

ACTION STEPS

- Create a birthday calendar so you don't have to rely on Facebook to remind you.

- Make a personal directory and share the contact information with mutual friends and family. You don't want to invade people's privacy, but if there are areas of overlap between your social circles, you've saved someone a lot of work.

- Start compiling a master to-do list. Put a check next to each item you complete.

The Healer Villager

The One Who Makes You Feel Better

*Healing is a matter of time, but it is sometimes also
a matter of opportunity.*

Hippocrates

There are myriad ways a healer can be part of your village. This might sound basic, but the healer is someone who can make you feel better. Of course, this can take any number of forms. For example, when a friend was sick, she asked everyone in her village whom she considered to have a great sense of humor to send her funny articles and clips of comedy sketches. The people who thoughtfully curated an assortment of jokes, humorous articles, and videos to make her laugh were healers. This was a small way we could make her feel cared for. Think of the ways you try to help others. Is it a form of healing? Have you ever cooked for someone? Preparing a meal or even baking cookies is a small way to help a person feel better. In short, there are countless ways to help someone heal, and we are going to explore a few options in this chapter.

A healer doesn't have to cure someone or fix what is broken in their life. The healer is there to lift their spirit and ease their worries. My best friend and I say to each other, "I may not be able to fix it, but I'll walk with you through it." This means that we know we'll be beside each other through big and small events. Having someone who can acknowledge the issue you're facing and stand by you is healing. This isn't always easy for me to practice, because instinctively I want to fix the problem.

I met one of my dearest friends in college. At this transitional period in my life, she helped me express my emotions. I watched how she helped other friends in need and realized she's quite intuitive. When I am trying to understand the why of something—like "Why did I react that way?"—this friend can get to the heart of the matter. This isn't fixing the problem but helping me understand it. In many cases, there is no fix.

I like being there for others, and I understand that it takes a special kind of heart to be able to practice this type of acceptance. You might be saying, doesn't the healer display the same qualities as the accepting villager? Yes, there is overlap, but the healer also has other qualities. In fact, being a healer can be a temporary role. Think about the traditional healer, a medical professional. They usually aren't a daily fixture in your life; they are there to try to heal you when you're sick. Also think about the qualities of a doctor or nurse. After spending way too much time being poked and prodded in medical facilities, I can tell you that a medical professional's bedside manner is vital to a patient's recovery. Sometimes people can't bring someone along with them when undergoing medical procedures or treatments. Being frightened and alone is a scary combo. My nurses made me feel cared for and listened to, and that was essential in my healing. As I mentioned before, because I was alone during so many medical procedures, I found myself turning to my digital village and making short videos to keep others updated on my progress, but I was probably subconsciously searching for a healer villager. When people saw my post, some reached out as cheerleaders, but others helped me heal. They distracted me with jokes, sent home-cooked meals, and showed up in other wonderful ways.

When I was going through IVF, I relied on an acquaintance who—quickly turned into an invaluable friend—because she had also had gone through IVF and knew how to help me. This person was like a one-woman support group and knew exactly when to reach out. If you find yourself helping someone who is going through a similar experience to yours, you are displaying traits of the healer villager. In other cases, an entire support group can serve the role of a healer. That said, sometimes when you go to a support group, you might unearth painful memories, in which case you might not feel better right away. There were times when I logged on to the IVF support group when I felt saddened by others' stories and felt vulnerable sharing mine. But this was all helping me heal, because I was addressing a challenge in my life.

Some secondary villages are healing groups. If you're part of a secondary village that was constructed when someone became sick, you can think of the entire group as healers working together. But let's explore how we define the word *healing*. Then we will answer questions, take quizzes, and reflect on a healer's role. Get ready to take out your notebook, and let's start talking about the ways we can locate a healer and become one ourselves.

What Does the Healer Villager Look Like?

Before we address what role the healer might play in your village, we can take a moment to reflect on how we define the word *healing*. Let's do a quick exercise to help us get a better understanding of the word!

EXERCISE

How Do You Define Healing?

- *When you hear the word* healing, *what are the first words that come to mind? Please write as many words as you can think of. Once you've done that, rank the words in order of importance to you.*

- *Write a short reflection on each word and address why you chose it.*

- *Isolate the top three words on your list. Why were those the chosen three?*

Remember, the beauty of these exercises is that they are just for you. This means that you can be completely honest when writing. It can sometimes be difficult to be truthful with ourselves, but try your very best to do so.

I included a ton of words in my own list, but the top three are *patience, comfort,* and *compassion.* Next I will show you how I see these as vital characteristics for a healer.

Patience

Patience is an essential quality for someone who takes on the role of healer. Even if they're a temporary fixture in your village, they should never make you feel rushed to heal. This person is there for as long as you need them. Growing up with a sibling who has special needs, I learned the art of patience, but there were times when Michael tested it. For instance, something like a bulb being out in our Christmas lights can really upset him, and we have to spend substantial time and emotional energy to calm him down. Moments like these are daily occurrences, and even the most imperturbable person in the world will occasionally find themselves losing their cool with Michael. Every time I lose it, I feel bad afterward. I know Michael has taught me about patience, but it wasn't easy to stomach. I remind myself that we are all imperfect beings, and I have to give myself grace.

Another aspect of my life where I have to maintain patience is behind the wheel. I wouldn't say I have road rage, but I can get very upset with other drivers. To help me maintain my composure, I play music while I drive.

The time when I had to really sit still and wait was when I was undergoing IVF. I also had to let go during this process. Although I did everything you could possibly do to be healthy during this period, I still couldn't control my thyroid and had to take a break. I desperately wanted to be a mother, but I also knew that my body had endured all it could. When I took a break, I was patient as I let myself heal. As I write this, I've learned that waiting and being patient were the best ways to heal myself. Once I took a pause, I was able to see how exhausted I was and how much I needed to recover. And that perhaps it wasn't the right time in my life to become a single mom.

Comfort

In essence, a *comforter* is one who can soothe. As a child, I was comforted by my stuffed bunny, Fluffy. Studies have shown that children who sleep with stuffed animals are better at self-soothing as adults. I'm not advocating for adults to start bringing stuffed animals into their beds (but if you do, more power to you!), but I want you to find what comforts you. This can be as uncomplicated as a cup of tea or a morning meditation. Although these comfort items or practices aren't healer villagers, they are healing rituals that can enable you, in small ways, to serve as your very own healer. But do you have a person in your life who also offers the same feeling? The person who can listen to your problems and make you feel heard and seen? These are a few traits of a healer.

Compassion

There is an entire chapter in this book dedicated to being a consciously compassionate person, but I also find *compassion* to be a healing word. Identifying how a person needs to be helped and healed is the true test of compassion. Serafina Ferrara, my great grandmother, and her husband, Salvatore, immigrated from Italy and started Ferrara Pan Candy. You might know this candy company because it was they who invented the classic candy, the Lemonhead. Although I never met my Nonnie, I learned about compassion from her. Years ago, I was able to track down a video of an interview of her. She was a respected female entrepreneur, which wasn't the norm for that time, and she was being interviewed about her company's success. She was a generous woman, someone who gave free cookies to any child who entered the shop. Every story my family tells about her is full of her kindness and philanthropy. In this grainy interview, where I clung to every word she spoke because I had spent years longing to meet her, she talked about her need to give back. In broken English, she said that if she had bread, and someone else needed it, she would give it away before taking it for herself. She said she wouldn't be able to sleep at night if she didn't help others.

That was a sampling of attributes you might want to have in your healer village. You might have another idea of what a healer looks like, and that's okay. This is space for you to define the healer in your village.

What Role Does the Healer Villager Play?

When we think of a healer, we often think of a doctor—a person who can fix what is wrong with us. This is not necessarily true of a healer villager. No one should expect someone else to solve their problems, no matter how good a friend they are. However, healer villagers *can* help a friend work through or think through their problems. Just as everybody has a different reason for going to the doctor, everybody has a different reason for why they need a healer villager. You might not realize it, but we all seek out forms of healing. Booking a massage, sitting in a sauna, taking a night to yourself, or walking with a friend are all small ways that we work to heal what "ails" us.

Once we recognize how we heal ourselves, we can identify how we might help heal others. Everybody has certain things that bring them comfort, and we can use these to provide healing. If you have a friend who doesn't like to talk much, a long conversation about their problem might only give rise to more anxiety, but bringing them their favorite coffee is another gesture of thoughtfulness.

When one of my friends lost her sister—who left behind two young children—I asked my friend's mom what I could do to help the family and my friend specifically. She said, "I saw you two on the couch, when you were watching the kids play. I noticed you held hands, and that was enough to help heal my daughter in the moment." She wanted me to know that sometimes the smallest things mean the most. For instance, when someone hugs you when you're upset, and you feel like you can let go and cry. Has that ever happened to you? It's happened to me a lot. We are all emotional, but we might find ourselves devaluing and underestimating the power of emotions. We can't bottle things up; we need to feel and process our emotions to survive. When we offer our love to help heal others, we should also be vulnerable. I know that isn't easy for people. However, being there for someone in a small way is better than not being there. Show the people you love that you care about them.

How Can I Be a Healing Villager?

Before you can heal others, you should first understand how to heal yourself. A healing villager can't be expected to heal others if they aren't feeling their best. Self-care is often associated with expensive spa treatments and time-consuming meditation practices, but it can be as easy as taking a minute or two out of your day to jot down things you're grateful for, or tuning in for an episode of your favorite TV show.

Self-Care Rituals

Watching TV or a Movie

Okay, okay, I know a lot of you probably think that watching TV or a movie is a passive way to partake in self-care. Some of you were probably raised like me and were told to limit your TV consumption. Today I say you won't understand the feel-good movie category until you don't feel good. I believe watching a comedic film or even a TV sitcom can heal you. I love watching *Friends*, and whenever I'm upset about something, putting on an old episode makes me feel better. I believe in the benefits of comfort TV.

Electronic Detox. Do Not Disturb

Yes, I did just tell you to watch TV to feel better and now I'm telling you to detox from screens. No, I'm not trying to drive you crazy. I do believe there's a time to consume television and other media, but there is also a time to put it away. I'll confess that I find myself losing large chunks of time mindlessly scrolling through social media, when I could have been reading a book or cleaning. I think we should allot time to detox from the endless world of social media and take a break from electronics.

Your Own Healing Ritual

I have a friend who loves to take a shower or a bath when she's feeling stuck, creatively or otherwise. She finds this to be a healing ritual. I find taking a walk to be healing. I love wandering through gardens or going on a gentle hike. Spending a few minutes in nature is wonderfully healing.

Calling Someone or Making Plans

If you're feeling bad about yourself, it's hard to make plans with others. However, seeing friends is a vital part of a well-rounded self-care routine. Sometimes I don't want to go out because I don't feel like I look like my best self. Maybe my face is a little puffy or I don't feel like I have the right outfit, but every time I quiet that inner voice and go out anyway, I always feel much better. When I go out and spend the evening laughing, I realize how much I needed it, and it shows me that we all need human connection. Sometimes, though, if we don't have the energy to go out, a call or text can also do the trick.

Reading or Crafting

I'm an avid reader and can easily spend the day immersed in a book. When I feel the need to do something creative, that's when I decorate—my idea of crafting—where bits and pieces of any holiday personality are placed throughout the home. Both reading and crafting are activities that I can do on my own. I am able to heal myself by putting myself in another mindset.

Retail Therapy

Confession: I really love shopping. Does that make me materialistic? No, it makes me human. I don't have to buy anything fancy. Even buying a pack of gum makes me feel better. I'm not a big online shopper; I think interacting with people in a store is probably more healing for me. Again, I love being social and will take any opportunity to chat and meet new people. And self-care can be as simple as creating a change of scenery in your own home. So you might want to pick up something that creates a sense of serenity. For example, I love candles, so burning a scented candle is a quick way to lift my spirits.

Journaling

A daily journaling practice is an excellent way to process your emotions on paper. If you're upset about something, you can work out a lot in the journal. Every few months I reread my journal and can recognize patterns of behavior that I'd like to address. Some might think that journaling is too vulnerable an act and fear that someone might read what they have written. If that sounds like you, you might want to write a letter or a journal entry and then destroy it. You don't have to hold on to the writing. The act of writing can help release emotions, and that is healing.

Now that we've discussed ways you can work on healing yourself, you might wonder how you can heal others. No, you don't have to go to medical school or to an institute that teaches people how to become energy healers. All you need to do is show that you care. It sounds straightforward, but as we discussed, everybody has a different definition of caring. Here are a few easy ideas for ways you can incorporate a healing practice into your everyday life. Take a moment to consider a few people in your life who might need extra comfort at the moment. Okay, do you have that list? Here are a few ways you can aid their healing.

Comforting Gift

A healing gift doesn't need to be anything expensive—merely something that you believe might bring your fellow villager comfort. When a friend of mine lost her husband, neighbors brought over food they thought she might like. Though these were small gestures, and they couldn't ease the pain she was feeling, they made her feel loved, supported, and cared for during an incredibly difficult time. She was comforted to know that she wouldn't have to worry about preparing food, and even more comforted to know that she was surrounded by a village of people who cared.

A Patient Ear

As a healing villager, you might feel a desire to solve all your loved ones' problems, but sometimes this isn't possible. Listening to somebody, in person or otherwise, can be a powerful gesture that helps them to feel less alone.

A Hand to Hold

Though you might not be able to solve a person's problems, you can certainly help them navigate them. If a friend is going through a hard time, you can help them find a support group or try to connect them with people who have gone through similar experiences, so that they feel less alone. If they're overwhelmed, offer to take some manageable tasks off their plate. When a person is dealing with something particularly painful, it can be difficult for them to handle all the small duties associated with daily life, so asking what they need a hand with might be a relief to them. Keep in mind, however, that you shouldn't take on more than you can carry. You can't help anybody if you're overwhelmed.

These are a few ways you can help heal others. Personally, I try to live my life in service to others. I think this is why I started out as a nanny. The idea that I could help others and take part in their families' lives seemed like a job that nourished both me and others. I also felt this when I was running a company. After years of nannying, I had decided to change my career. At the same time, my father found himself bored in retirement and wanted to start a company. He asked if I could help him. It was the motivation I needed, and this began my career as the head of a now-woman-owned digital-content company. Making it a woman-owned business meant that I had to lovingly fire my father, and this has become a long-standing inside joke in my family. Of course, I enjoyed producing digital content, but the real joy was working with others to create a product. I thrive on teamwork, and now that we've talked about the final villager, the healer, I'm going to spend the next few chapters talking about getting off the bench and being part of the team.

I'm going to close this chapter by sharing a small but meaningful moment in my life. During the holiday season after the worst of the COVID-19 pandemic had passed, I was finally able to see my extended family. This time, we hugged a little longer. We didn't do anything besides sit around and tell stories. Listening to these stories was healing to me. I'll admit that there were times when I didn't appreciate these family get-togethers, but this year it wasn't just special, it was restorative. Being with my village in real life was what I needed to get through the following exhausting year.

GUT CHECKS

- Describe a time during which you felt helped by someone.

- When was the last time you helped someone?

- Do you feel better after you see certain people? Why?

ACTION STEPS

- Send someone who is having a bad day a link to a humorous video, article, or even perhaps a song. People love to hear a song reminding you of them!

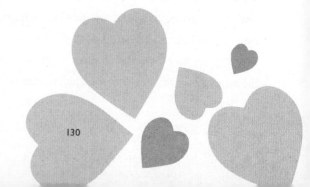

- Buy or make postcards and send handwritten notes to your friends, family, or someone who could use a smile. Even a "cheer you up" text.

- Order a meal for someone who is stressed out. There are so many websites and even apps to make this easy!

How to Be a Compassionate Villager

The Empathetic One

*Generosity is the most natural outward expression of an
inner attitude of compassion and loving-kindness.*
His Holiness the Dalai Lama

I don't want to sound as if I have the world's biggest ego, but I see
the qualities of all these villagers in myself. Throughout the years,
I've been accepting, dependable, a cheerleader, a communicator,
a healer, and an organizer. Don't hate me, though! I can also rattle
off a list of the villagers in my life who also encompass all these
roles. You can make fun of me, but this reminds me of the ending

of *The Breakfast Club*. (By the way, loving John Hughes movies is nearly a requirement when you grow up in the Chicago suburbs.) If you haven't seen that film, I'm about to throw a major spoiler your way, so you might want to skip ahead to the next paragraph. At the end of the film, the students who spent their Saturday detention sharing intimate stories discover they have a lot more in common than they had originally thought. After they broke down their barriers and let different people into their lives, each of them walks away from the day realizing they shouldn't be labeled as one type of person. They weren't just "a brain, an athlete, a basket case, a princess and a criminal."[1] This movie tried to deconstruct labels that are often placed upon high school students, and to show the audience that when pretense is stripped away we are all alike. We have to give one another a chance.

As I stressed earlier, you don't need to search for six separate villagers who display these qualities. You can find these qualities within yourself and others to create a working village. This isn't just a list that you can check off as you go. If you do that, you won't be seeking people in your life for who they are, but what they can do for you. You don't order villagers like you order a pizza! You need to find people who can help and be compassionate, and who are capable of being in a relationship that mutually enhances both of your lives.

Let's talk about the word *compassion*. We can play different roles in various communities, but compassion is the essential quality each villager must possess. Compassion isn't passive but active, meaning that like any art form, we need to find ways to practice it. How do we practice this? Here is a great example. I have a friend who lives in New York City who takes a walk with her neighbor every Friday afternoon. They stroll down to a local bakery and pick up treats for their families. The bakery offers a free cup of coffee with every purchase, but my friend and her neighbor had always passed on this free offer. You might wonder why I'm sharing such a small detail with you, but bear with me, I promise it's an important one! One day when they were walking toward this bakery, located on a bustling city street, there was a homeless man sitting on a small crate and asking for any spare change. Her neighbor walked toward the homeless man, who was bundled in blankets to keep warm, and asked him if he wanted a cup of coffee. He smiled and replied, "I'd love one."

"How do you take your coffee?" her neighbor asked.

The man proceeded to tell her how he liked his coffee, a basic question he might not have heard in a long time. The neighbor ordered her pastries, accepted the free coffee from the bakery, and handed it to the homeless man along with a muffin. My friend admitted that she had passed this homeless man several times—he had become a fixture in their neighborhood—but she had never offered him anything. She realized that she could have been providing him with a hot cup of coffee every Friday for weeks, yet this thought had never occurred to her. Her neighbor was actively practicing compassion, and witnessing this inspired my friend to be more mindful. The key to practicing compassion is not big gestures or self-sacrifice but being conscious of what you can do to help.

I know I'm not perfect, but for the past few years, I've been trying to actively practice compassion every day. IVF tested this for me. There were weeklong stretches where I felt tired and queasy after egg retrieval. For those of you who haven't been through IVF, it's an emotional rollercoaster. You prepare by filling your body with a cocktail of hormones to bring multiple eggs to maturity. The entire process was a physically and emotionally draining experience for me, and when I was going through it, I had to learn to be compassionate with myself, which is the first step toward being compassionate with others. After all, how can we understand how to be kind to others, if we cannot be kind to the person we know the best—ourself?

I understand that compassion is something of an abstract concept and can't be learned overnight. That's why I've tried to synthesize compassion into six main traits—which correlate with the six villager roles—making the art of compassion one that anybody can fully engage with. When you embody one or more of these roles, you will, without even realizing it, become a more compassionate person to yourself and others. Of course, compassion, like any skill, takes time to master. Be patient and gentle with yourself and others as you build your beautiful village.

Which Villager Are You?

As you were reading about the qualities of the villagers highlighted in the previous chapters, you might have already recognized yourself. Maybe you realized that you're the cheerleader. (I mean, didn't you already like twenty people's social media posts today?) But perhaps you now want to foster aspects of another villager within yourself. You can use the gut-check questions paired with the action steps to achieve that goal. Maybe you've never felt put together enough to host an event, but you've often served as a conduit between people. You want to engage that organizer persona, so you decide to organize a neighborhood cleanup. While you rake leaves in a town park, you can be cognizant that all these roles are malleable and that you can be different things to different people. The key, however, is balance, and you must acknowledge that you can't serve in all roles at once. The perfect village is about harmony. Your role might look different in each group, but each village should remain fully populated even if some villagers are fulfilling multiple roles.

As you try on new roles in the new village you're crafting or the existing one you're joining, it's a good idea to keep a journal chronicling your experiences. It's a great way to track your progress and to be candid with yourself. Speaking of being honest with yourself, there are times when you should do a gut check and see if you're capable of taking on a role as a certain villager. Sometimes being part of a community means knowing your limitations, and it's much better to let somebody know that you can't serve in a certain capacity than to let them down later. Here's a quick exercise to help you practice being a compassionate villager and learn how to be compassionate with yourself. Take out your journal!

Villager for a Day

Make a list of all six villagers. For the next six days, try your best to practice the qualities for each one—a different one each day. Keep a journal of what you do to nurture the characteristics of that specific villager and how it makes you feel. Hint: You might want to start by practicing one of the action steps from the chapter for that villager.

Now you've actively tried to be different villagers. Some roles probably felt natural, and others might have taken you out of your comfort zone. This is okay. Be compassionate with yourself. Even if one of the roles felt instinctive, sometimes that role might change. For instance, if you asked them months ago, the people in my various villages might have called me the organizer. I love to socialize, and

I enjoy the intellectual stimulation that comes with lively conversations. Yet these past months, I've been too drained to play the part of organizer while stimulating my ovaries in that seemingly never-ending IVF process. I was in a nesting phase. Then I went through the stage where I had to reconcile with myself that I couldn't go on with the process. During that period of my life, I retired from my role as an organizer. As with anything in life, sometimes we need breaks, at times you may need to take a sabbatical from your role in the village. This means all the people who had cast me as the organizer in their networks now had to find a replacement, but that doesn't mean I had to leave their villages entirely. Instead, I could fill new roles! I'm the perennial accepting villager and cheerleader, and I knew I could be both to others even while fully immersed in other things of priority.

I discovered I couldn't be an organizer in the traditional sense. I found myself organizing lots of events online and soon found that I was depleted, so I did a gut check. Based on that, I decided to pause my organizing efforts. I realized that it is important to practice active compassion with myself.

Remember, you have the power to decide who you want to be, but you also have the power to decide who you *don't* want to be, and the power to recognize who you *can't* be. We must know our limitations or we won't be effective villagers. Remember the gut-check questions in chapter 1? The ones where I asked you to write two lists—the people who depend on you and the people you depend on? Maybe some of you have a long list of the people who depend on you and a much shorter list of the people you can depend on. If you have an asymmetrical list, with way too many people depending on you, it would benefit you to learn the art of saying no. Remember to prioritize helping yourself before you help others. If you are a constant helper, take a break and learn to accept help.

Maybe you were someone's dependable villager, but now you don't feel as dependable. When I was working long hours trying to start a small business, my work obligations hindered my ability to be a present and dependable friend. Though I was still there to help my friends when they were in crisis, there were events I had to miss, and my time was often limited. Many adults find themselves in these types of situations. The best way to increase dependability is to pay attention to time management and study how you use your time. Even if you're clocking a sixty-plus-hour workweek, you can still check in with a friend in need or send over a meal. Small acts mean so much. It's imperative that you make it clear to a fellow villager when you need to redefine a relationship. While it's important that you set your own boundaries, you also don't want to leave somebody in the lurch. The best villages are ones in which members feel comfortable communicating their needs and expectations.

By now you might have noticed an ongoing theme in this book: being a villager isn't a role you assume all at once but a continual series of acts and conversations. Partaking in these small acts—centered around helping others—increases your sense of well-being and has the potential to be life-changing for others. Before you dive headfirst into village life, figure out what role you are going to feel best in. Keep in mind that each role can look different in various communities. So, which villager are you? And more importantly, which one do you *want* to be?

Can You Be Every Villager?

Every one of us has the potential to be every villager—but not all of them at the same time. When I'm in my family village, I play a long-established role. My family sees me as the cheerleader villager, while my cousin is the dependable one. But my group of friends might see me as their dependable villager. We all play a variety of roles in different people's lives, and understanding which role we play in various villages can substantially enrich our relationships.

Perhaps we could also call this chapter, "Which Villager Do You Want to Become?" Is there a part of you that you want to nurture? Remember, you can be every villager, but it might zap you of your energy. When I was taking care of my grandparents, I felt like I was all six villagers and then some. As a caregiver, you continually switch roles while tending to another. Countless caregivers wind up utterly depleted. There's a term for this: *compassion fatigue*, or caregiver burnout. You don't have to be someone's personal caregiver to suffer from this. Hospitals run workshops on this issue to equip their staff with the tools to navigate the mentally exhausting world of being a professional caretaker.

I have a confession. Despite once being employed as a nanny and later being a voluntary caregiver to my elderly grandparents, I used to feel guilty grouping myself with doctors, nurses, therapists, and other professionals who are often diagnosed with compassion fatigue. I felt that my job as a caregiver wasn't challenging enough to warrant having any symptoms, but this was far from the truth. When you come to another person's aid, you can feel fulfilled and loving, which is wonderful. But you can also feel overwhelmed, and this is okay. Feeling these negative emotions does not mean that you don't love the person you are caring for, it simply means that you are human too. Taking time to care for yourself should not feel like a guilty pleasure. It's a necessity when you are caring for others. After all, if you feel exhausted all day, you won't be able to perform to the best of your abilities.

Even if you have the ideal village, when you care for someone who is either in pain or unable to care for themselves, you can suddenly find yourself drowning in your own emotions. When that happens, you cannot just tread water endlessly; you must swim to the surface. If you don't, you won't be able to stay afloat. To make sure you aren't drowning, please do regular check-ins with yourself.

And here is something else worth recording in a journal: try keeping a sleep log. You can tell a lot about your mental state by your sleep patterns. Having good sleep hygiene is an essential facet of self-care that many people overlook, especially when they're busy. Getting enough sleep is hard when you're taking care of a newborn or an elderly person. I can't tell you how many sleepless nights I clocked when I was taking care of my grandparents. I'm sharing this with you not because I want to sound like a martyr, but because I want to warn you about taking on more than you can handle, and caution against the hazards of being a one-person village. Thankfully I was not a one-person village—my mom being their primary caretaker—but even thinking of her doing all that by herself is overwhelming! A deep emotional toll comes with caretaking. Even if you have the perfect support system, you can still feel emotionally overwhelmed, and compassion fatigue might surface. Don't expect that your villages make you immune to these emotions. Instead, lean on your people to help support you through them. These emotions aren't a dirty little secret. By sharing them with your villagers, you might feel much better. You might even find that they have felt, or are feeling, the same way, which can bring you closer together.

As with a good diet, and pretty much everything else in the world, the key to success is balance. Even if your life is unexpectedly chaotic and you feel balance is unattainable, be sure to continue the practice of gut checks. Always ask yourself how you are feeling;

don't wait for someone else to ask you that question. If you're too overwhelmed to answer, try to think of one task you could assign to someone else that would make your life slightly easier. Even having something as small as doing the dishes or going to the grocery store taken off your plate can give you room to breathe and figure out what you really need. Continually leaning on your village in small ways like these is often more beneficial than any big gesture. I also believe we all have the capacity to create effective companionship if we practice compassion every day. Even one small act of compassion to ourselves and others will help fortify the foundation of a village.

I truly believe we all have the inner capacity to be every villager, but that doesn't mean we should try to assume all these roles at once. The balance between what we *can* and what we *should* do is often a difficult one to achieve, and your role in a single village shouldn't leave you emotionally spent and incapable of self-care. Rather, it ought to strengthen you. The most important gut check you can perform is simply to ask yourself if your relationships are working, and if you feel that you are receiving from them a balance of what you provide.

How Can We Actively Practice Compassion in Our Village?

The other day as I was taking a walk, I saw a teenager muttering to himself as he stood outside a local coffee shop. I noticed a few people on the street walking away from him, but I realized that he was afraid of a dog that was outside the store and was searching for another entrance into the shop. I immediately recognized this behavior because I had seen my brother react similarly. When the teen realized there was a side entrance, he entered the shop, but he was quite unnerved by the experience with the dog, and I worried how the people inside might react to him. I decided I couldn't let him walk through the door alone, and I followed him in, ready to serve as his advocate. I stood in the line behind the teen, and fortunately he calmed down and ordered an iced tea. Even though I hadn't planned on ordering anything, I ordered a beverage and watched the teen safely exit. If the boy had acted out in the shop, I'd hoped to communicate to others why his behavior seemed erratic and to potentially de-escalate the situation. I had imagined constructing an impromptu village with the other customers, but thankfully it was not needed.

Since I was a child, I have been exceptionally aware of behaviors similar to those of my brother. However, you don't have to experience living with a special-needs sibling to be conscious of those who might need help. We can become more mindful of the people in our environment and try to put ourselves in their shoes, even if it's only for a second. I know the boy in the coffee shop might have frightened a few people because he didn't follow social cues and was muttering to himself. You're not a bad person if you distance yourself from people displaying similar behaviors. However, if you pause and think about what might be causing their behavior—in this case being unnerved by a dog—you can try to help others who might not be capable of helping themselves. You should never do so at the risk to your own safety, and boundaries are important too. This is why I chose to quietly follow the boy rather than approach him. I didn't want to further agitate him, nor did I want to put him or myself in a dangerous situation. I simply wanted to be ready to come to his aid if it looked like he needed it.

Years ago, when my Nana was home recovering from a broken hip and I was assisting her, a friend and her daughter come over for a visit. My Nana was an incredibly warm person who was full of life. Every night, no matter how much pain she was in, she had to have a coffee and dessert. This was a ritual, and for years both of my grandparents would entertain guests, sharing cake and coffee. As a kid, I thought it was a sweet (both figuratively and literally) way to end the day. On this night, when my friend and her daughter were visiting, I had to help my Nana walk over to the table. After I eased Nana out of bed and ensured that she was securely standing with the help of her walker, I watched as my youngest guest guided Nana out of the bedroom and to the dining room. I looked over at my friend and asked, "How did you teach her to be so compassionate and aware of a person in need?"

She said that her daughter had watched how adults treated her great-grandmother and was mirroring those behaviors.

Her daughter learned how to be compassionate by observing others' behavior. This reminds me of some of the best advice I gave as a nanny. Parents would ask how they could raise a respectful child, and what means of discipline best ensured this. Without fail, I'd tell them that children mirror our actions, and respectful children are raised by respectful adults. If children see adults practice compassion, they will do the same, and if children see adults act in a callous or rude manner, they will mimic this behavior too. The cliché that children are like sponges is true. The rules we set for our children mean absolutely nothing if we don't follow them.

I was lucky to be brought up by a mother who is the quintessential villager. She knows how to ask for help and has mastered the art of reciprocity. A few months ago, her neighbor, who also is one of her best friends and like a second mother to me, was recovering from surgery. My mother invited her to stay with her while she recovered. While I was at my mom's house, her neighbor needed to shower and was unable to do it on her own. I placed a shower chair in the shower and used the detachable shower head to help clean her. My sisters were shocked that I dared to engage in such an intimate activity with her, but I was unfazed. I thought back to how vulnerable my grandmother had felt, and I wanted Mom's friend to know that I was there for her. Without hesitation, I took what I had learned from caring for Nana and used those skills on behalf of another. It reminded me of my friend's daughter guiding my Nana from the bedroom into the kitchen. In these moments, my friend's daughter and I both expanded our village, providing care not only to our families but to those we saw were in need.

What I also recognized in the little girl was that she wasn't shy of adults. When I was a child, I was also unafraid of adults. I wanted to know what adults knew. As a kid, I felt like they held all the secrets to grownup life. I was taken with the perfumed older relatives who came over for family celebrations. As all the cousins played together, I'd sit with the adults, absorbing their conversations and trying to make myself a part of them. I'll always remember when my step-grandmother, who was affectionately known as Grandy Mitzy, came to visit. She was so glamorous to me. A socialite, she sparkled when she spoke, and she always commanded a room. Grandy Mitzy let it be known that she wasn't a fan of kids once they passed the adorable stage of babyhood. She was the opposite of Nana, a woman who had a lap filled with grandchildren and to whom I could tell anything. However, I made it my mission to connect with Grandy Mitzy.

When Grandy Mitzy came over I'd run up to her, while my more timid cousins would shy away. I'd ask Grandy Mitzy about her life, and she would tell me entertaining stories that I delighted in hearing. Why am I telling you this? I learned in my living room as a child that different people fill different needs. Nana was the grandma that I laid my head on. Grandy Mitzy, on the other hand, was the type of grandma who connected with kids almost in an adult way. She wanted mature conversation, and I was tickled to hear stories of glamorous adult life (even if they had to be edited to become PG-rated). Connecting with somebody is a beautiful thing, and no two people bond in quite the same way. As you're establishing your village, be conscious that the ways you connect with one member might be entirely different from the ways you connect with another. This doesn't mean that one relationship is stronger than another. Just like snowflakes, they're all unique.

GUT CHECKS

- When was the last time someone thanked you for helping them?

- How much time do you spend helping others? Be honest! Keep a journal for one week.

- How do you communicate with yourself when you are feeling overwhelmed? How do you communicate this to others? How do these methods differ?

ACTION STEPS

- While on a walk or even while running an errand, try locating one person who might need assistance. This could be a small act like helping someone reach something from a top shelf at a grocery store. The key here is to be aware of your surroundings.

- Try to keep a daily journal of ways you might help others. You might even set daily goals in the journal.

- Take five minutes out of your day to do a gut check. Ask yourself how you are feeling. Answer honestly! If you are feeling burnt out or displaying signs of compassion fatigue, reach out to someone.

What Happens When the Village Is Lost?

Rebuilding Your Village after Loss

Be the change you want to see happen.

Arleen Lorrance

In times of crisis, we often unearth our hidden strengths. This is also a time when we need our support systems the most. Ironically, it's during these periods in life when a village might be destroyed. For instance, when a certain chapter of our lives closes, we sometimes lose the characters who played roles in that chapter. This is especially true when we build our villages around other people's needs. Whenever we are tasked with starting over, we need to rebuild or reconfigure our communities. Yes, rebuilding has its challenges, but now that you have the template for constructing a village, you will have the tools to create a new one.

Although we've discussed this before, I must go back to the COVID-19 pandemic. I'll always recall how quickly our lives changed. In an instant, we lost many of the villages that had kept our world together. This period also catapulted folks into significant change. It was during this time that I decided to permanently move out of Chicago and sell my business. Those were big, life-changing decisions, and I was certainly frightened, but with an increased understanding of the fragility of life, I knew I had to embrace uncertainty in order to find true happiness. I also knew I would have to rely on old circles while I designed new ones.

Moments of vulnerability are often scary and isolating. However, they can also serve as opportunities. We can use our most vulnerable times to engage in self-exploration and try to understand what it is that we really want and need, and what aspects of our lives are inhibiting us. The period when I was taking inventory of my life brought me a moment of extreme clarity. I realized that the "single-girl" village that had kept me going for over a decade had disappeared. Everyone had left Chicago, and I felt like I was the last one standing. This was something that had been happening for years, but I had been trying to ignore it. One by one, everyone in my Chicago village had either left for the suburbs or joined a new support system when they got married and had a baby. Yes, there was a skeleton crew, but the group was no longer satisfying me like it had in the past. It was then I realized I had to rebuild.

This may happen several times throughout your life, as you transition from one period to another. You might have picked up this book because you're at one of these transitional stages. We experience numerous transitions in life—from graduating college and establishing yourself in a post-college community to becoming a new parent. Major life changes often indicate the need to rebuild or restructure a community.

Rebuilding a village isn't easy. Although I knew I needed a change, I was exhausted from the intensity of keeping my company afloat. As I mentioned before, I brought in a business consultant, and although their recommendations strengthened the business, we never expected a pandemic to take over our world. I knew I had to do something different, but I wasn't ready to pivot.

The idea of changing my life overwhelmed me, and I longed to stay in neutral. I'm sure we've all felt this way before. It's at times like this, when everything is in flux, that you might wish you were back in your old life. Just like we watch TV shows from our youth to recapture our feelings from those years, we often find comfort in the familiar. So when I was changing my life, I also wanted my old friend circle back. Of course, this wasn't an option. I had to make bold moves and big changes. When a business associate (spoil alert: she's who I ended up selling my company to) asked me what my end-game was for my company, I spit out the words, "I think I want to sell my business." This was something I had been internalizing, but it was the first time I had vocalized this thought. Even I was shocked hearing these words pop out of my mouth. Immediately I told myself selling a business wasn't a sign of defeat but a realization that I had to take another path. I knew I had done all I could with my company. It needed to be taken to the next level, but I didn't know how to scale the business. This was when I suggested we merge companies.

Merging is one of the best ways to grow a business, and it's a concept that can also apply to villages. When you merge networks, you make them stronger. The only downside to this is that sometimes we lose people in the process. We might also lose our identity as a villager. For instance, in the business world, I was used to being the CEO and the founder. When I merged the business, it was no longer mine. Even though I had a position of leadership, it wasn't my company. The once small and mighty village that I had created was now a large and powerful company.

When a village is lost, you can construct even stronger and more powerful villages. Once you discover what you need and how you can be part of it, you can create multiple support circles that will enhance your life and the lives of the people around you. In this chapter we will talk about rebuilding, and merging our support networks, as well as finding our bearings in these restructured villages.

How Do I Rebuild a Village?

It's lonely without a village. Although America had been suffering a loneliness epidemic for years, the pandemic highlighted the harmful impact of social isolation. Since 2020, there have been countless articles on the insidious impact of loneliness. Having friends is essential for our mental health. According to one academic medical center, "Adults with strong social support have a reduced risk of many significant health problems, including depression, high blood pressure and an unhealthy body mass index (BMI). Studies have even found that older adults with a rich social life are likely to live longer than their peers with fewer connections."[1] Of course, we don't have to be "friends" with everyone, but we do have to be friendly and work well with them. Being part of a community is a positive life experience, and also good for your health!

So what do we do when we feel alone? How do we dare construct a village when everything has been lost? Even if you need a new village because you're moving to a new city for a dream job, you are still far away from your old village, and that sacrifice can be quite a challenge. When I moved to Los Angeles, I was living out a dream, but I also felt lonely. I'd look at families sitting at other tables in restaurants and wonder what my family was doing at that moment. This was tough, yet I was doing something I wanted. What about people who didn't chose to lose their village?

A good step, when we feel like things are at their worst, is to take a moment to journal. Writing is a healing modality and a great way to process our thoughts. I understand that when when we are overwhelmed, we might not have the energy to write much. You want to know what I do when I'm overwhelmed? I make lists! Here's a short list of questions to answer to help you rebuild what has been lost.

Rebuilding the Village

- Do you need a primary or secondary village? Or both?

- What roles are missing in your village?

- What are looking to replace in your village?

Okay, you did it! It's not an intense list of questions but they do help you figure out what you need from this new community. Now, I want you to take a break and reflect on the villages that you were part of in the past. Perhaps until you picked up this book, you hadn't realized you were part of a network. However, we've all been part of villages throughout our lives, and we need them to go forward in life. I know rebuilding is a challenge. As I mentioned, I recently moved and was terrified over how a single person would be perceived in a family-friendly suburb.

Now we're going to work on the second part of the exercise. Keep your notebook out and answer this question: Can you name three people you know who live close by? They can even be casual contacts.

Good. Now look over the names. When I was doing this exercise, I included my real estate agent on that list. Yes, my mom does live close by, but I was looking to find people who would help me to be more social outside of my family village. I wanted to find new friends in a familiar place. That said, you can jot down any name you want, but just because you put those names on paper doesn't mean you have a village. However, you will use this list as a place to start building connections. Remember in chapter 3 when I asked you to create a list of people who are there for you and then cast them to be in the village? You can go back to that exercise and use it to recast this new village.

Can I Incorporate Old Villagers into My New Village?

Sometimes we don't want to rebuild a village in the same place we were living. Sometimes we need to make a big change. This was how I felt when I was living in Chicago. It's ironic how you can live surrounded by countless people yet feel so isolated. When my Chicago village disappeared, I didn't want to rebuild one in that city. Instead, I wanted to relocate. In short, I had outgrown my life in Chicago. Although it wasn't easy to admit, once I did so, everything seemed to fall into place.

Some people feel like they've failed when they move back to the town they grew up in, but I felt like I was finally home. When I moved to a house in my old hometown, it was the first time in decades that I felt like I belonged. Don't get me wrong, I enjoyed my life in the city, but there was something about the familiarity of a place I knew so well that made me feel welcomed and loved. At the same time, it had been ages since I'd lived in this town, and my old friends had established their own lives and villages. This was the new-girl moment as I tried to fit into my friends' villages. Would I just insert myself into their groups or start my own?

The hard truth: I was the odd woman out. I was living in the suburbs but was not married and didn't have kids. My friends hung out as couples or as families, and here I was, the single gal from the city trying to fit into suburban life. Within a few weeks of living in my new home, I was invited to a block party thrown by my neighbors. We all live off an alley, and the residents of my block refer to themselves as the Alley Cats. This was almost like being invited into an instant village. Although I was excited about the invitation, I wondered how they would perceive me. I wasn't like anyone else on my block, because these folks seemed to live similar lives to my friends' suburban existence. Again, I was the singleton and worried if I would be accepted.

My fears were unfounded. An hour after I'd met the Alley Cats, everyone was cheering me on when they heard about my IVF journey. They also began to chant "village," and at that point, I knew I had found my people. I honestly felt a big sense of relief. I was worried that I wouldn't be accepted, and here I was, feeling so loved by my new neighbors. Since then, I have seen the Alley Cats in action. We check on each other's homes when someone is out of town, and other such dependable actions. What can I do for them? How can I be helpful for them and be part of their village? I reciprocate. Being in this village doesn't mean that I need to be around my neighbors and helping them out every day, but I should be there in the background, and they do the same. As we watch out for one another, there's an awareness that we're a part of something, and we're there to answer that call.

While creating a new village, I was also revisiting old circles—ones I hadn't been part of in decades. How do we work within pre-existing villages that we're returning to? Again, the first thing to ask yourself is how you can be of help to the people in your community. Try to be proactive. Many people are introverts and this doesn't come naturally to them, so remember that there's no shame in taking small steps. I've highlighted three steps you can take to incorporate old villagers into your new village:

- **Be honest.** If you had to restructure your village and create a new one, explain why this happened. Honesty is the first step in proper communication.

- **Know your needs.** Explain how your needs changed and why you still want these people to be part of your life.

- **Accept others' actions.** If you're merging a village and someone doesn't want to be part of the new one, you must respect their decision. This doesn't mean you won't be upset by it, but you can't control others' actions.

Remember, you don't have to give up your role in a village if you move away. You can still be "there," but in other ways. I have a bittersweet story about how someone who passed away is still part of her young daughter's village. It's a heartbreaking yet heartwarming story. My friend's sister died of thyroid cancer. A single mom, when she was diagnosed she was given only a couple of months to live. She had two young girls, so she bought gifts for her daughters for every single occasion in their lives that she'd miss once she passed away. She even put together a break-up kit for the first time their hearts were broken, and for celebratory moments from graduations to birthdays to parenthood.

We talk about how we need a village to raise a child. My friend and the grandparents raise the kids now, yet the mom is still present in her thoughtfulness. Throughout their lives these girls will have reminders of how important they were to her and how loved they will forever be. As I am fond of saying, we have to let love in. If we do, we will always have a community.

How Can I Be Part of a New Village?

In the past year I've made lots of new connections but I'm still trying to create new villages in my community. Although I've established myself in my friends' villages by being present and seeing what the group needs, I'm reaching out to neighbors and trying to join community groups. Working to establish relationships tends to get harder as you age because you inevitably have more responsibilities, and your life is more structured. So, maybe joining a wine club or a running club isn't high on your priority list. You might realize that you've shelved your social life, and it's hard to reactivate it.

This means you can find yourself sitting at home on Saturday night, scrolling on social media, and then begin to think you aren't living your best life. This is a toxic pattern, and I know I'm not the only one who does this. If this sounds like you, it's time for action. Finding the right people for your new village will be rewarding.

As you search for new groups, try to go out of your comfort zone. Note that you can't find a village unless you are willing to work with others. Joining a village is a commitment, and you should take it seriously. If you're reading this book because you burned your old village down, I hear you. We all have times when we can't deal with our old communities and might accidentally (or intentionally) set them "on fire." Know that no matter how bad it seems, if you do reach out to former members of the village, they could be receptive. Sometimes you need to toss your ego aside and apologize or have a conversation that addresses the dissolved village.

GUT CHECKS

- Name a time when you felt you lost a village.

- Name a time when you had to rebuild a village.

- How did the new community compare to the old one? Did you take on different roles in the new village? Why?

ACTION STEPS

- Host an event where at least two people don't know each other. This could be casual, like a happy hour or a potluck dinner.

- Say yes to at least one invitation in the next month. It can even be a virtual event. It doesn't have to be a big event—it could be a talk at the local library—but it should be an opportunity where you'll meet new people.

- Look through your contacts and find one person you haven't spoken to in a while. Invite them to have coffee.

Depending on Yourself and Your Village

Recognizing Your Role in the Village

The expectations of life depend upon diligence; the mechanic that would perfect his work must first sharpen his tools.

Confucius

It's so much easier to write all this out than to enact it in your daily life. Every day, I take steps to build and maintain my villages, so I know that embarking on this journey can be really challenging. This is why the first step you ought to take is to serve as your own self-sustaining village. Depend on yourself. In small ways try to heal yourself, to organize your life, to serve as your own cheerleader, to communicate with yourself, and to accept the times that you fall short. This might seem overwhelming, but you probably do these things every day without realizing. Each morning, when you get out of bed, it is your cheerleader motivating you to take on the day. When you take a few deep breaths to calm yourself after a stressful situation, that is your inner healer at work. When you make plans with a friend, your organizer is in action, helping you maintain the relationships that matter to you. Oftentimes, the person you are hardest on is yourself. Give yourself credit for all that you do to nourish your needs. In areas you feel you could be more supportive, try to identify which inner villager would be best to invoke.

The key to healthy villages is healthy villagers, and this starts with you! Before you go off and build the beautiful communities that I know you will, take a deep breath and work to fortify yourself. Becoming your own village doesn't mean that you won't rely on the networks around you, but it does mean that because you can rely on yourself, you won't ever have to settle. In becoming your own support system, you are learning your own value and giving yourself the space to create positive and gratifying villages that work with you. In essence, being your own village provides you with choice. Never feel pressured to join a group, and don't pressure another person to join yours. Instead, join a village because it will enhance your life, and invite others in because you believe it will do the same for them.

A friend of mine, Becky, lost her job and had to relocate to a new city to find work. Moving to a place where she didn't know a soul, she felt isolated, especially considering that her job was entirely remote. She realized that she was lonely, and she invoked her inner healer and inner organizer and decided to adopt a puppy. She befriended neighbors at the dog park and began building friendships. When Becky couldn't rely on outside villages, she supported herself by making choices that benefited her. Something as joyful as adopting a pet brought her love and comfort. When I recommend that you be your own village, I'm not suggesting that you must carry all of your burdens alone—only that you listen to yourself and do your best to fulfill your own needs as they come. After all, if you cannot provide support to yourself, how will you help others support you, and how will you support others?

How Can I Be a Villager to Myself?

Like anything, acting as your own ally takes time and practice, but there are ways to nurture your inner villager. In chapter 9, we talked about self-care rituals and how being your own villager is an act of healing. However, there are any number of ways you can be a villager to yourself. I like to say that being your own villager isn't just a self-care practice, it's a self-soothing practice, which means it helps you feel comfortable with yourself.

You have the capacity to make yourself feel better. You know yourself better than anyone else does, but sometimes you might not recognize patterns that hinder self-care. For instance, are you the type of person who doesn't like to do things for yourself? Do you feel guilty when you take a day off? Or buy yourself something nice? I know I'm guilty of stopping myself from fully enjoying good news in my life, and as I said before, when positive things happen my best friend says she's the one who will be happy for me. But why do I act like that? Why am I not a cheerleader for myself when I love cheering on others? I created a quiz to see if I'm being a good villager to myself. There will be another quiz in this chapter that assesses if we're a good villager to others, but first, let's see how we treat ourselves. Don't worry, this is a quick exercise and there are only three questions. Take out your notebook and answer honestly.

Are You Being a Good Villager to Yourself?

- *How do you self-soothe?*

- *How do you care for yourself?*

- *How do you take inventory of your mental, physical, and emotional needs?*

You may wonder what "taking inventory" means. Taking inventory of your needs can happen in various ways. You can reflect on your mental, physical, and emotional state. You might want to answer the above question by writing down the words *mental, physical,* and *emotional* and placing a number next to each. Ten would mean you are doing the best mentally, physically, or emotionally. One would mean that you're in need of some serious self-care. Also, be gentle when answering that question. I know I'm hard on myself. For example, when I don't go for a long walk (I try to do two hours a day!), I can believe that my physical needs are zero, which is far from the truth. This means we shouldn't try to focus on how we feel this minute but should try to focus on how we feel in general. Maybe today isn't your best day, but you have something fun planned for tomorrow. You should factor the past few days into this self-evaluation.

To help you figure out how to be a better villager to yourself, here are a few tips:

Tips for Being Your Own Villager

- Be present.

- Be honest.

- Challenge yourself to continue to grow.

- Be curious.

- Always question.

After an intense year, I reconnected with a friend from childhood. We both needed emotional support at that time, which strengthened our bond. It didn't take long to discover we were more than friends. For years, I had been my own "single-gal" village, and I was happy, but as we grew closer, I realized I had been missing companionship. I was enjoying myself in a way that I hadn't in many years.

I'll admit that in previous relationships, I constantly asked my friends for advice about the guys I was dating. I wanted to hear their opinions to validate my impressions of these men. I needed to hear multiple opinions because I believed that would help me decide if the person was a good fit for me. In fact, one time when I was dating someone and he went to the bathroom, I asked the waitress what she thought of him. Yes, I needed that much reassurance that I was with the right person. Though that relationship ran its course and purpose, it showed me something very imprtant: partnership is something I want, and for so long I had convinced myself I didn't. Even dating takes a village and building tools! And I have to take my own advice now.

As I learned to become my own villager, I realized that I could be my own cheerleader and accepting villager. I learned that I *wanted* to be my own support system in this regard. Although I believe in the concept of a village, there are times when you're enough, and you can make those decisions. When we age, we often develop a tendency to edit our instincts and think about past experiences that might have been painful, and this can stunt our actions. Listen to your gut and trust yourself. Once you're able to do that, you will have more substantial and secure relationships with the people you invite into your community.

I've also learned that when we have to pivot in life, it can be exciting. I thought the endgame was having a baby and being a single mother, but maybe it was obtaining the peace of mind that I *can* do so, by freezing my eggs. I was fortunate enough to freeze time, and my eggs will always be thirty-five years old. I'm ready to be a mom, when the time is right. On my time! And right now, it is not.

How Can I Show Others I Want to Be Part of Their Village?

The first step before becoming part of anyone's village is to reflect on your potential role. Think about ways you might be able to help them rather than ways they can help you. Now that you've done the work in this book and answered the gut checks, addressed the action steps, and taken several exercises and quizzes, you should have unearthed new beneficial qualities within yourself. Perhaps you haven't thought of yourself as a cheerleader, but you see the small ways you bring joy to your life. Feel confident enough in what you offer. However, also consider what you think that community might *need*. I'll acknowledge that I've long been curious about human behavior and how groups work well together. When I was in school, I'd look at the various cliques and think about what that group of friends had in common. I would also wonder what I could bring to that group if I wanted to befriend them. I know this might sound like strange behavior for an adolescent, but I was always observant.

When I went away to college, I used these skills when I was trying to figure out which sorority to join. I wanted to find one where I'd fit in, so I tried to figure out what the common denominator was within each group. One of the reasons I picked my sorority was because the women in that house had similar values to mine. Although they didn't look like me, they *felt* like me. And to this day, I'm still best friends with three women I met when I was in college. I often reflect on how certain decisions impact the trajectory of your life. If I hadn't joined that sorority, I would not have met these women who quickly became my primary village. No matter where any of us live, they will always be my North Star.

As you can see, I am getting back to the word *values* again. I don't believe you should only befriend people who have the same values as you do, because it's important to have an array of people who bring different opinions and perspectives to your life. You don't want to only surround yourself with people who think like you do, because it would be rather dull and wouldn't challenge you. It's important to respect others' values, even if they are different from your own.

Listen, I'm human and I know that it's hard not to judge others, especially if we question their values. Still, be mindful of others and try to see things from their perspective.

Even if you meet people who share your values, it doesn't necessarily mean that those values will translate to new friendships. You might also fear being rejected by the group, which is entirely normal. That said, try not to limit yourself because of fear. I believe feeling uncomfortable is vital for our growth. My advice is to be brave and be comfortable with being uncomfortable. If you can do that, you can create a village.

As outgoing as I am, I still get nervous when I am embarking on something new. I serve on a highly regarded hospital board in Chicago. At the first board meeting I attended, once the presentation started—from the researchers to the physicians—I was instantly impressed by the wealth of knowledge in the group. I scanned the room and realized I was the youngest person there. Then I also realized that I was seated next to some of the most successful people I'd ever met. This was a moment of utter intimidation, even though everyone was pleasant to me. To quell my nerves, I recalled my dad saying, "If you're the smartest person in the room, you're in the wrong room." While I felt out of my depth, I realized that this was an opportunity for me to learn from others, challenge myself, and ultimately make a difference for a cause I believe in.

Let's do an exercise now. Please take out your notebook again. Think about the last time you were part of a group of new people. It could be the first day on a job, the first day of school, or your first meeting with a book club. It could even be a situation where you knew the people, but you hadn't seen them in a long time. Now I want you to answer these three questions to assess how you react in social situations.

EXERCISE

Nice to Meet Yourself—Getting to Know YOU

- *What emotions do you feel when you're asked to attend an event where you don't know many people?*

- *How have you navigated these types of social events in the past?*

- *Write one good memory from a party. Why did you choose that memory?*

Now that you've answered these questions, you will have a better understanding of how you interacted with people in the past. This will serve you when you begin to form your villages. We don't often stop and ask ourselves deep questions. Earlier in the book I said that I don't like small talk; I like real talk. This concept doesn't just relate to chatting with others, but also when talking to ourselves. We need to sit down and ask us ourselves some real questions. Once we can do that, we can have deeper relationships with both ourselves and others. If we take the time and care to reflect on previous situations, we will see that we've done a lot of the hard work before, and we can learn from it. Self-reflection is essential.

So, how can you be a part of someone's village? Realize what you can offer them. Now, you don't *have* to be this focused when seeking out a group. There is merit in jumping into a group and seeing where you land. You do want to be flexible. For instance, you might want to be a cheerleader, but they are looking for an organizer. Maybe you can do both! You're probably tired of me talking about being a nanny, but that was a major part of my life, where I learned the importance of being part of a support system. Of course, since I was a hired villager when I was a nanny, my role was a bit more defined, which certainly made it easier. However, the longer I spent with a family, the more my role developed, and sometimes I was more than the hired dependable villager. I was also the child's cheerleader.

It's not always easy to join a new village, but the tools in this book can apply to any village-building situation. It doesn't matter what changes are happening in your real life—this book can be your guide to help you with those moments.

How Can We Depend on Our Village?

As I said in the beginning of this chapter, you have to depend on yourself first before you can depend on anyone else. In fact, now that we've reached the end of the book, you should already have a pretty good idea of why and how you should depend on your village. However, I wanted to reiterate that we need to begin with ourselves. If we aren't able to take credit for our lives in small ways, we won't be able to help others. We also don't want to take advantage of another's kindness, or let someone take advantage of our kindness. If we take

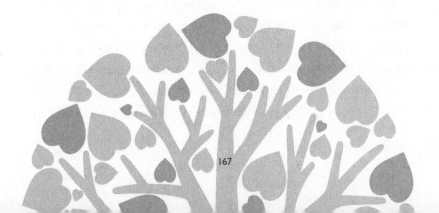

steps to be our own villager before we become someone else's, we understand the impact and importance of that role.

In this book, we've talked about the subtle signs that we are utilizing a community properly or accidentally abusing it. We also talked about the six essential villagers we need to form a complete village. Finding these people will help us create a balanced world for ourselves. We don't want to overly rely on them, and by isolating these six traits, we can utilize the positive traits of a villager rather than focusing on the negative. My goal is that you stop thinking of one of your villagers as the "chronically late" villager and start thinking of them as the cheerleader, or the accepting villager, or whatever trait shines through. Many of us focus on the negative aspects of a person's personality, and hopefully by isolating one of these six traits that they do have, we can see that everyone has the potential to be an active member of a community.

I've confessed to my love of reality TV and the show *Friends*. It's funny, but once I isolated these characteristics in the members of the villages I belonged to, I began to see these traits in various TV characters. You can observe various villages on TV and see how each character has a certain role in that community. If you pick your favorite movie or TV show, I bet you can easily place each character into one of these six roles. Of course, TV isn't real life (not even reality TV), but it's fun to see how we can study characters through this lens.

Now that we have the tools, we are ready to go out and start our villages. Remember to be compassionate when you begin your journey. Enjoy the experience of creating these new villages in your life. If you ever feel lost, you can repeat the exercises in this book. I would like to leave you with one more exercise. You can use it to check in with yourself if you're questioning your place in one of your networks, or if you want to see if the village is working. It's always good to pause and reflect on how your village is functioning and whether anyone might be unhappy in the circle, including you!

Village Checkup

- How long have you been part of this community?

- How exactly do you feel nourished by this support system?

- How do you nourish this village?

These are three questions you should think about when you're trying to assess whether the village is working for you. As I said before, reflection is key to helping us discover what is working in our lives. Stopping to question our actions is the only way we can grow and understand ourselves. Once we embark on that journey of questioning, we can better practice self-love and begin the process of creating a village with others, prepared to spread compassion and love.

Now that you have the directions to the village, it's up to you to go and find it! Remember: Let love in. Ask for help. And find your people.

GUT CHECKS

- When is the last time you felt part of a community?

- Who or what is missing from your village?

- What's one thing you expect from your new village?

ACTION STEPS

- Reread your answers to all the exercises, quizzes, questions, and gut checks in the book.

- Make a list of the actionable findings from what you wrote.

Start today by identifying your first villager.

Acknowledgments

To my family—you are the beats of my heart and the breath to my life.

To my friends—thank you for lifting me up, your arms around me, and your inspiring kindness.

To Devra—you took a chance on me and stood by my side through every obstacle, delay, and challenge. Thank you for being my sun.

To Alison—thank you for your outstanding collaboration, your sweet friendship, and your immeasurable talent. Without you, this book would not have been possible.

To Steve Allen—my surrogate Dad, the one who sees me for me; thank you for showing me how to truly, deeply, and purely love.

To the Beyond Words publishing team—thank you for believing in me and seeing the soul of this book. You made my dream come true.

Notes

INTRODUCTION

1. "Loneliness and Social Isolation Linked to Serious Health Conditions," Centers for Disease Control and Prevention, last updated April 29, 2021, https://www.cdc.gov/aging/publications/features/lonely-older-adults.html.
2. John Bowden, "Michelle Obama Says Upcoming Memoir Shares the 'Ordinariness of a Very Extraordinary Story,'" *The Hill* (Washington, DC), June 22, 2018, https://thehill.com/blogs/blog-briefing-room/news/393754 -michelle-obama-says-upcoming-memoir-tells-ordinariness-of-a.
3. Mayo Clinic Staff, "Friendships: Enrich Your Life and Improve Your Health," Mayo Clinic, January 12, 2022, https://www.mayoclinic.org /healthy-lifestyle/adult-health/in-depth/friendships/art-20044860.
4. Emma Rubin, "Elderly Loneliness Statistics: Adults Report Feeling More Isolated in 2021," updated February 17, 2022, ConsumerAffairs, https:// www.consumeraffairs.com/health/elderly-loneliness-statistics.html.
5. "Windy City Nanny: the Series," Florence Ann Romano, 2021, https:// www.florenceann.com/web-series.
6. Pete Seeger, "The Old Left," interview, *New York Times*, January 22, 1995, https://www.nytimes.com/1995/01/22/magazine/sunday-january-22-1995-the -old-left.html.

CHAPTER I

1. Florence Ann Romano, "How to Build Your Village," *The Windy City Nanny*, episode 11, October 22, 2019, YouTube video, 9:14, https://youtu .be/1yOyotXepkA.
2. Florence Ann Romano, "Village Building Chart," August 15, 2019, https:// www.florenceann.com/resources.
3. Nick Tate, "Loneliness Rivals Obesity, Smoking as Health Risk," WebMD, May 4, 2018, https://www.webmd.com/balance/news/20180504/ loneliness-rivals-obesity-smoking-as-health-risk.
4. Gary Chapman, *The Five Love Languages: The Secret to Love That Lasts* (Chicago: Northfield Publishing, 1992).

CHAPTER 2

1. Amanda Mull, "The Pandemic Has Erased Entire Categories of Friendship," *Atlantic*, January 27, 2021, https://www.theatlantic.com/health/archive/2021/01/pandemic-goodbye-casual-friends/617839/.

CHAPTER 3

1. Mayo Clinic Staff, "Social Support: Tap This Tool to Beat Stress," Mayo Clinic, August 29, 2020, https://www.mayoclinic.org/healthy-lifestyle/adult-health/in-depth/friendships/art-20044860.
2. Fox 24 News Now, "Single Motherhood Through IVF | Fox24 News Now," September 9, 2021, YouTube video, 6:47, https://.youtu.be/0QuaQ5ny3oM.

CHAPTER 4

1. Florence Ann Romano, "When Your Parents Watch Your Kids," *The Windy City Nanny*, episode 2, August 21, 2019, YouTube video, 8:41, https://youtu.be/GECk7GPG1n0.
2. Florence Ann Romano, "'Let It Flow, or Let It Go' Chart," August 21, 2019, https://www.florenceann.com/resources.
Shonda Rhimes, "Drowning on Dry Land," *Grey's Anatomy*, season 3, episode 16, directed by Rob Corn, aired February 15, 2007, https://www.netflix.com/watch/70158951.
Jenny Bicks and Cindy Chupack, "Splat!," *Sex and the City*, season 6B, episode 6, directed by Julian Farino, aired February 8, 2004, https://www.hbomax.com/series/urn:hbo:series:GVU2cAAPSJoNJjhsJATt6.
3. Bill Walsh, Don DaGradi, and P. L. Travers, *Mary Poppins*, directed by Robert Stevenson (1964; Burbank, CA: Walt Disney Home Video, 2013).

CHAPTER 5

1. Erin de Cespedes, "Choosing an Emergency Contact—It Matters," Nolo, accessed March 4, 2022, https://www.nolo.com/legal-encyclopedia/your-emergency-contact-it-matters.html.
2. Family Caregiver Alliance, "Caregiver Statistics: Demographics," 2016, https://www.caregiver.org/resource/caregiver-statistics-demographics/.
3. Tia Slightham, interview by Florence Ann Romano, Instagram, June 22, 2021, 31:11, https://www.instagram.com/tv/CQbXWR3D3_0/.
4. Michelle Cottle, "Who Will Take Care of America's Caregivers?" *New York Times*, August 12, 2021, https://www.nytimes.com/2021/08/12/opinion/caretakers-elderly-home-health-aides.html.

CHAPTER 7

1. Nina Spears, interview by Florence Ann Romano, Instagram, November 22, 2021, 22:35, https://www.instagram.com/tv/CWlbOJWDtYU/.

CHAPTER 10

1. John Hughes, director and writer, *The Breakfast Club* (1985; Universal City, CA: Universal Pictures).

CHAPTER 11

1. Dana Sparks, "Mayo Mindfulness: Friendships Enrich Your Life and Improve Your Health," Mayo Clinic, September 4, 2019, https://newsnetwork .mayoclinic.org/discussion/mayo-mindfulness-friendships-enrich-your-life -and-improve-your-health/.

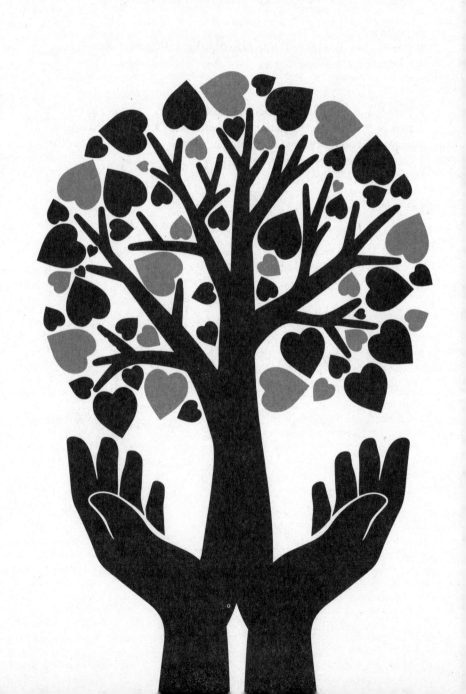